Kindly Donated
by
Dr Stafford

ABC OF
PLASTIC AND RECONSTRUCTIVE SURGERY

ABC OF
PLASTIC AND RECONSTRUCTIVE
SURGERY

DAI DAVIES FRCS

Consultant Plastic Surgeon, West London Plastic Surgery Centre,
West Middlesex University Hospital, and honorary senior lecturer,
Royal Postgraduate Medical School, Hammersmith Hospital, London

with contributions from

M BRIGGS, H CHENG, M POOLE, J J PFLUG,
J RAYNE, ROGER SMITH, C M WARD

Articles published in
the *British Medical Journal*

Published by the British Medical Journal,
Tavistock Square, London WC1H 9JR

First published 1985

British Library Cataloguing in Publication Data

ABC of plastic and reconstructive surgery
1   Surgery, Plastic
I. Davies D M   II.   British Medical Association
617'.95   RD118

ISBN 0–7279–0122–2

Printed in Great Britain at the University Press, Cambridge
Typesetting by Bedford Typesetters Ltd, Bedford

Contents

The illustration on the back is taken from *Ophthalmodouleia das ist Angendienst* by G Bartish, Dresden 1583.

Introduction

The term plastic appears to have been introduced in the early nineteenth century. Graefe used the term "rhinoplastik" to describe a method of reconstructing the nose using skin from the forehead, and Langenbeck used "Organische plastik" to describe a branch of surgical reconstruction using living tissue as opposed to artificial prostheses. Thus plastic surgery became that part of surgery concerned with the living replacement of parts and usually involving the movement of skin either by making it more mobile or by a transplantation using skin grafts (Zeis 1838).

Today a plastic surgeon's repertoire extends beyond the skin to include surgery on blood vessels, nerves, tendons, muscles, cartilage, and bone. As these procedures become more complex, often requiring a team approach, the term plastic and reconstructive surgery is being increasingly used. Today's plastic surgeon will spend about 30% of his time on surgery for congenital abnormalities, 30% on traumatic problems, 30% on oncological problems, and 10% on cosmetic improvement.

The earliest written accounts of plastic surgery in the West are by Celsus (25 BC-AD 50), who in his book *Chirurgia Curtorum* described surgical operations to correct congenital cleft lips and mutilations of the nose and ear. Undoubtedly Jews did reconstruct the foreskin. There are also at least two accounts of possible reconstruction of the foreskin in the Bible, but these references may refer more to giving up circumcision. Later, in Roman times, the operation was performed because it was considered a disgrace to appear in wrestling schools (Palaestra) with the glans uncovered.

The art of reconstructing noses and ears had, however, been described in the classical text on Indian surgery, *Susruta Samhit* (circa 600 BC), which originates from the four Vedas texts of divine Hindu knowledge. In the second text Lord Dhanwomtni, a physician to the gods, gives specific descriptions of surgical tools and techniques.

In 1794 in London there appeared in the *Gentleman's Magazine* a letter to the editor on the "Indian method" for total nasal reconstruction. The letter was probably written by an English surgeon, Cully Lyon Lucus, who worked in Madras, and it describes with illustrations an operation to reconstruct the nose of a bullock driver performed by a man of the brickmaker caste near Puna. This operation, using a midline forehead flap, is still used today to provide skin cover for a nasal reconstruction. The article revealed for the first time to the Western world the secrets of this procedure, held by several Indian families, who passed them from one generation to the next.

Having read this article Joseph Carpue, surgeon to the York Hospital in Chelsea, in 1816 published an account of two successful operations for restoring a lost nose using the same technique.

Nasal reconstruction was also developed independently in Europe. In the fourteenth century the Branca family of Sicily used a forehead flap reconstruction very similar to the Indian method. In 1430 Antonius Branca experimented and used a flap of skin from the upper arm to cover the nose, and this method was popularised and finally recorded by Gaspare Tagliacozzi of Bologna in his book on plastic surgery published in 1597, *De Curtorum Chirurgia per Insitionem*. The so called Italian method was a six stage nasal reconstruction using skin from the inside of the upper arm.

In the early nineteenth century techniques of plastic surgery developed under great general surgeons such as Dieffenbach, who undertook important observations on the design and blood supply of skin flaps for nasal, eyelid, and lip reconstruction. He was succeeded in Berlin by von Langenbeck, who developed techniques for the closure of cleft lips and palates. The first world war provided a major impetus to the development of techniques in reconstruction, particularly the transfer of large areas of skin around the body and more major operations on the face. The tube pedicle, consisting of two random flaps joined together, was introduced in 1916 simultaneously by Sir Harold Gillies and Vladimir Filatov, an ophthalmic surgeon in Russia. Gillies, who trained as an ear, nose, and throat surgeon, later became the first plastic surgeon to be appointed to a London teaching hospital (St Bartholomew's).

The introduction of the local anaesthetic cocaine in 1884 and its use in nerve blocks by Holsted together with the introduction of general anaesthetic allowed for better operative conditions. Gillies was able to extend the use of his own skin flap though the improved anaesthesia provided by Dr Magill, who developed and introduced the endotracheal tube and intratracheal insufflation of anaesthetic gases, which allowed many advancements in technique in the head and neck.

In the past 25 years there have been tremendous developments in the understanding of the blood supply of the skin and its underlying structures, which have allowed skin to be transferred around the body in one stage procedures, which are far more predictable and safe. With the introduction of the operating microscope plastic surgeons have been able to join together blood vessels of smaller and smaller dimensions. Thus severed digits and limbs can now be replanted, divided nerves repaired more accurately, and composite tissue blocks (free flaps) moved around the body and their blood supply reanastomosed to local vessels.

The development of these new reconstructive techniques has allowed plastic surgeons to work much more closely with colleagues from other disciplines, and patients with cancer of the head and neck, with cleft lips and palates, and those with compound trauma of the limbs are now all likely to be looked after by multidisciplinary teams.

The techniques developed in reconstructive surgery also provide a means of altering or improving a person's appearance. In 1583 George Bartish designed a clamp to remove excess skin in the upper eyelid. In 1887 Roe of Rochester, New York, described an endonasal approach to reduce the size of the nose, but Jack Joseph (1865-1934), a Berlin surgeon, is considered to be the father of the rhinoplasty operation. In 1912 Eugine von Hollanden described the first anterior incision to undermine the facial skin to perform a face lift. There is no doubt that there are patients who may receive therapeutic value from cosmetic surgery; and whatever else cosmetic surgery does it demands the highest surgical technique. Therefore if for no other reason it should be retained in the training and practice of plastic surgeons. The comment of Tagliacozzi remained as applicable today as it was in 1597: "We bring back, refashion and restore to wholeness the features which nature gave but chance destroyed not that they may charm the eye but they may be an advantage to the living sole, not as a mean artifice but as an alleviation of illness, not as becomes charlottans but as becomes good physicians and followers of the great Hyppocrates. For although the original beauty of the face is indeed restored yet this is only accidental and the end for which the physician is working is that the features should fulfil their offices according to natures decree."

CLEFT LIP AND PALATE

Incidence

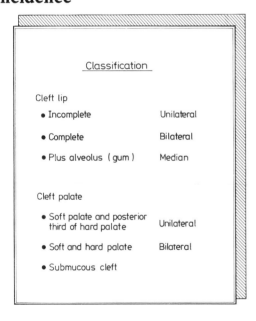

Classification

Cleft lip

- Incomplete   Unilateral

- Complete   Bilateral

- Plus alveolus (gum)   Median

Cleft palate

- Soft palate and posterior
  third of hard palate   Unilateral

- Soft and hard palate   Bilateral

- Submucous cleft

Cleft lip occurs in one in every 750 live births, affecting boys more often than girls and the left side more often than the right. Cleft palate affects one in every 2000 live births, and girls are affected more often than boys. In half of all cases a cleft of the lip and palate occur together. Other cases are roughly divided between cleft lip and cleft palate alone. Overall, the incidence is slowly increasing and it is the most common congenital abnormality of the head and neck. The aetiology of cleft lip with or without cleft palate is multifactorial. It is determined by a genetic predisposition involving several genes plus intrauterine exogenous factors. Cleft palate alone is genetically and embryologically distinct. When parents who are both unaffected have one child with a cleft lip the risk of a subsequent child having a cleft lip or palate is about 5%, rising to 9% if there are two affected siblings. When one parent and one child are affected the risk is about three times greater than in the normal population. Exogenous factors, including the use of thalidomide, phenytoin, or anticancer drugs during pregnancy, or possibly folic acid deficiency, have been incriminated in the formation of facial clefts. In about 3-5% of cases cleft lips and palates are associated with congenital syndromes affecting other parts of the body.

Embryology

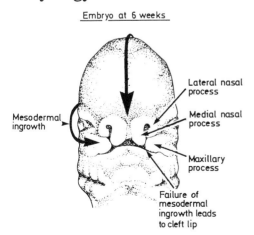

Embryo at 6 weeks

Lateral nasal
process

Medial nasal
process

Mesodermal
ingrowth

Maxillary
process

Failure of
mesodermal
ingrowth leads
to cleft lip

The cleft deformity is established in the first six to eight weeks of pregnancy. Two causes have been postulated: (1) a failure of fusion of the maxillary processes with the nasal processes; or (2) incomplete penetration of the mesoderm into the epithelial membranes of the medial and lateral nasal processes and maxillary processes. When the epithelial membranes break down this results in a cleft of the lip or gum, or both.

The palate develops from two shelves from the inner aspect of the maxillary processes, initially separated by the tongue, which with age descends and allows the two shelves to fuse in the midline by the end of the eighth week of pregnancy, joining from front to back. If the shelves fail to fuse, or the mesoderm fails to penetrate fully, a cleft palate forms.

Cleft lip and palate
Management

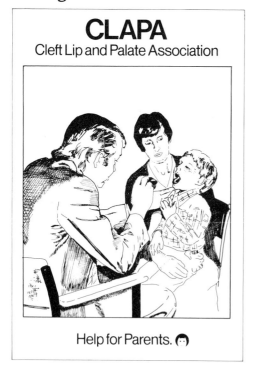

CLAPA
Cleft Lip and Palate Association

Help for Parents.

Patients with cleft lip and palate will require medical supervision from birth through to adult life and the attention of many different specialists including plastic surgeons, orthodontists, oral surgeons, ear, nose, and throat surgeons, paediatricians, speech therapists, and child psychiatrists. Obviously these patients are best looked after under the umbrella of a combined team, where all or most of these specialists can be seen in one visit as necessary, making treatment more convenient for the patient and permitting an interchange of ideas between the members of that team. Such an interchange may lead not only to an improvement in the management of the individual patient but also to improvement in the overall management of other patients with cleft lip and palate.

Few things can be more devastating for a mother than to go through a normal pregnancy only to give birth to a deformed child. A member of the team should always be available to see any such mother as early as possible so that she can have some of her anxieties dealt with and be reassured that help is at hand. Of equal help at this time can be a counsellor of the Cleft Lip and Palate Association (CLAPA). This is a self help organisation run by parents of children with cleft lips and palates, who are able to counsel other parents in this difficult initial period by visiting them in hospital and also by advising them about such problems as feeding. CLAPA has regional groups throughout the country, usually associated with plastic surgery centres. Its headquarters' telephone number is 01-405 9200 x 256.

Repair of cleft lip

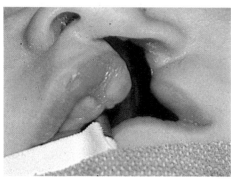

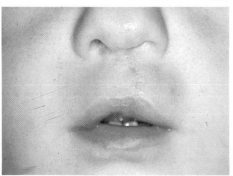

Modern techniques of repairing cleft lip appreciate that the deformity affects not only the skin but also the orbicularis muscle, the underlying maxilla, which tends to be hypoplastic, and the nose, in which the septum is deviated and the alar cartilage is hypoplastic on the side of the deformity. The emphasis is to correct as many of these deformities as possible at the initial operation, and as a result each surgeon tends to have his own modifications of one or other of a few standard techniques. My own personal technique at the initial operation consists of:

(1) Repair of the nasal layer of the anterior alveolar cleft.
(2) Correction of the nasal deformity by repositioning the alar cartilage.
(3) Muscle dissection on both sides of the cleft to reconstitute the orbiculris oris muscle.
(4) Millard rotation advancement to repair the skin.

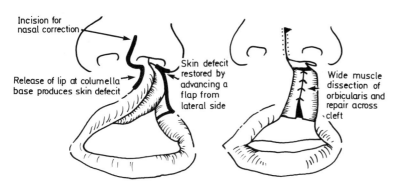

Incision for nasal correction

Release of lip at columella base produces skin defect

Skin defecit restored by advancing a flap from lateral side

Wide muscle dissection of orbicularis and repair across cleft

Most surgeons still depend on the rule of 10 for assessing the time of closure—that is, the child should weigh 10 lb (4535 g) and have a haemoglobin concentration of 10 g/dl; these usually occur together when the child is about 10 weeks old. This delay allows the lip and nose to increase in size for more accurate surgery and the child to withstand safely a longer operation. There are some surgeons who undertake lip repair (usually a simple lip adhesion) within the first 48 hours after birth. This obviously gives great psychological support to the parents but requires a neonatal surgical unit with experienced anaesthetists and does not give the conditions for a more radical closure; either final closure or additional procedures may consequently be required later.

Repair of cleft palate

Original cleft deformity

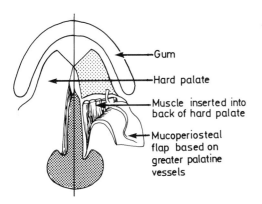

- Gum
- Hard palate
- Muscle inserted into back of hard palate
- Mucoperiosteal flap based on greater palatine vessels

Muscle dissected free and repaired in midline

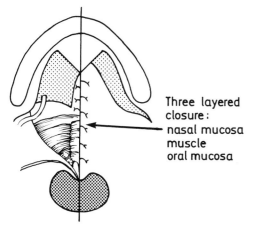

Three layered closure:
nasal mucosa
muscle
oral mucosa

Modern techniques of palate repair appreciate that the major abnormality, apart from the cleft, is that the velar muscles in the cleft are abnormally inserted into the back of the hard palate. The soft palate being a muscular organ, the velar muscles have to be dissected free and repaired in the midline of the reconstructed soft palate. In addition, radical dissections, particularly the stripping of the oral mucosa and periosteum off the hard palate, may result in scarring and interference with the growth potential of the maxilla, which can later result in collapse of the palatal arch and a flat face. Surgery for the hard palate is therefore becoming less radical, and indeed some surgeons now close only the soft palate at the initial operation, leaving closure of the hard palate to be performed much later.

Cleft palates are now being closed much earlier and should be repaired between the ages of 6 months and 1 year. This gives the child the correct anatomical and physiological apparatus with which correctly to mimic sounds that he hears, which is the start of speech development.

Clefts of the palate may be associated with considerable underdevelopment of the mandible, resulting in the tongue prolapsing into the oropharynx and thus interfering with breathing—the Pierre Robin syndrome. This may delay surgery until the mandible has caught up in its growth. Submucous cleft palate is a condition in which superficially there does not appear to be a cleft of the palate but in which the uvula may appear bifid and a notch on the midline of the back of the hard palate may be palpated. The essential defect is that the muscles, as in a cleft of the soft palate, are inserted incorrectly into the back of the hard palate. Patients with this condition usually present with either regurgitation of food or difficulties in speech and require a repair of the muscle sphincter of the soft palate.

Loss of hearing

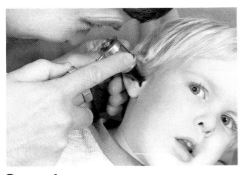

Children with cleft palates show a high incidence of loss of hearing. Two thirds of patients aged between 5 and 13 are affected. The muscle tensor palati arises from the eustachian tube and inserts abnormally into the back of the hard palate in patients with cleft palates. This may be a reason for drainage problems of the middle ear occurring, leading to an increased incidence of middle ear infection and thus to conductive hearing loss. Ear infections should therefore be treated promptly and the ear drums inspected regularly. Any loss of hearing may have a deleterious effect on the development of speech. Treatment is by decongestants, antibiotics, and myringotomy.

Speech

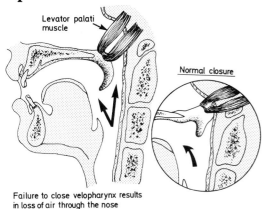

Levator palati muscle

Normal closure

Failure to close velopharynx results in loss of air through the nose

Roughly three quarters of children with a cleft palate will eventually speak normally. The palate, being a muscular organ, moves upwards and backwards during speech and completes a sphincter with the lateral and posterior walls of the oronasal pharynx, stopping air going up the nose and diverting it out of the mouth. In children with repaired cleft palates the sphincter may not be completely occluded and air will therefore escape up into the nose, producing nasal escape. Children with nasal escape may try to compensate for this by abnormal movements of the tongue to stop loss of air. This and abnormal dentition will produce errors in articulation. Abnormalities causing nasal escape can be corrected by surgery, but articulation can be corrected by the patient alone. The ability to talk normally depends on: the surgical success of closing the soft palate and producing a competent muscular sphincter; the presence of normal hearing; the intelligence and motivation of the patient; and parental encouragement to speak correctly.

Cleft lip and palate

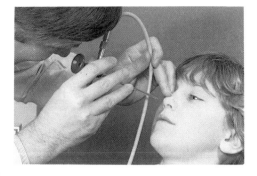

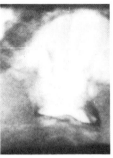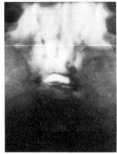

Basal view of palate showing incomplete closure of sphincter.

Children who do not speak correctly are usually referred to the speech therapist, who makes the initial assessment. The speech therapist can alter articulation patterns and give the patient exercises to improve movement and coordination of the palate using artificial speech aids. Most severe cases of nasal escape may well require surgery, with about 20% of patients with cleft palates undergoing pharyngoplasty.

The assessment of the palate includes an oral examination of the soft palate to see, on movement, whether the levator muscles have been successfully repaired or whether they remain inserted into the back of the hard palate and whether oronasal fistulas are present. X ray examination of the palate may be undertaken but requires cinefluoroscopy and includes lateral and basal views of the sphincter. Lastly, a nasendoscope may be passed down the anaesthetised nose and the palate viewed from above during normal speech. The exact position and size of the gap between the soft palate and the rest of the sphincter may be seen and the appropriate type of pharyngoplasty designed for the patient. There are many different designs of pharyngoplasty to achieve the desired effect of diverting air into the oral cavity. It is important to note that in a patient who has just undergone pharyngoplasty the voice may initially appear to have changed very little; it takes a trained ear to appreciate that the nasal escape has indeed been cured. The patient, if he had abnormal articulation patterns before surgery, will then need to learn correct articulation.

Later procedures

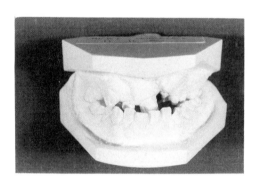

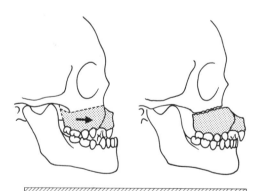

Timing of procedures	
0- 3 months	Repair of cleft lip
6-18 months	Repair of cleft palate
4 years	Preschool "touch up" of lip
6- 9 years	Pharyngoplasty for nasal escape
9-11 years	Alveolar bone graft Orthodontic procedures on secondary dentition
15-18 years	Maxillary osteotomies Adjustment of tip of nose and rhinoplasty

The orthodontist is an important member of the cleft palate team, who, as a specialist dentist, acts firstly as the archivist. Using plaster study models he can record the initial deformity and follow the growth of the palate from birth to maturity, recording the effects of operative procedures. Secondly, by the use of lateral skull radiographs, he can analyse the growth and development of the jaws and maxilla and advise his plastic and oral surgical colleagues on the exact physical abnormality in terms of size, shape, and position for bones of the developing face. Thirdly, he is called on at various times, from infancy onwards, to manipulate the teeth and jaws into better alignment by the use of appliances. For orthodontics to be successful the secondary dentition must be healthy, and this can be helped by enthusiastic oral hygiene from an early age and the addition of fluoride—in domestic water, in toothpaste, or in tablets.

In some patients disturbance of growth may be so great that orthodontic treatment alone will not suffice. Such patients may have considerable hypoplasia of the maxilla, extreme malocclusion of the teeth, and occasionally an overdeveloped mandible. Once the exact abnormality has been diagnosed major osteotomies can be performed by an oral surgeon, usually when growth of either the maxilla or mandible is considered to be complete, to realign the facial bones. These major movements of the facial bones permit correction of the dental occlusion and also improve the harmony of the face.

Late Cosmetic Surgery

Small adjustments may be required to the lip scar, including the production of a nice smooth vermilion. Apart from any osteotomies that may be required, the most common cosmetic abnormality in these patients may well be the nose. Many patients who are now reaching adulthood have not had primary correction of the nose, principally because it was thought that any early surgery might interfere with its growth potential. The nose slumps down on the side of the cleft, and the septum is deviated. At about the age of 16 a correction of the tip of the nose is undertaken together with surgery to the septum, which may be combined with formal rhinoplasty.

I thank my colleagues of the combined lip and palate clinic at the West London Plastic Surgery Centre, West Middlesex University Hospital.

CRANIOFACIAL SURGERY

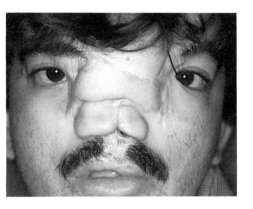

Craniofacial surgery is concerned with surgical correction of problems affecting the skull base, orbits, and upper face. These anatomical areas, in particular the skull base, were until recently a kind of "no man's land" that did not fall within the province of any particular surgical specialty. In recent years multidisciplinary teams have been formed to deal with problems in this difficult area. Because these problems are not common and management is difficult craniofacial surgery is performed in only a few centres with surgical teams treating sufficient numbers of patients to maintain the required level of skill. The conditions treated in this way fall into three main groups: congenital anomalies, tumours, and trauma.

Congenital anomalies

Congenital craniofacial anomalies

Simple vault craniosynostoses

Craniofacial synostoses – Crouzon's syndrome
                          – Apert's syndrome
                          – Others

Orbital displacements

Encephalocoele

Miscellaneous – Treacher Collins syndrome
             – Hemifacial microsomia
             – Others

The craniosynostoses are a group of disorders in which one or more of the sutural joins between the cranial bones becomes prematurely ossified, impairing the growth of the skull that takes place in a direction at right angles to the suture. This may lead to a deformity of the cranium (and eventually to deformity of the facial skeleton in some types) and, in some children, to mildly raised intracranial pressure, which may be harmful. Many cases of simple craniosynostosis do not require surgery and are managed expectantly, but in those where surgery is necessary it is usually done fairly early in infancy to obtain the best results in terms of subsequent growth. The surgical procedure in some of these conditions needs to be carried into the anterior skull base and upper face.

Types of craniosynostosis

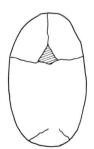

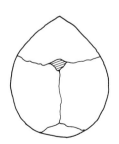

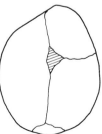

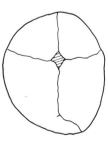

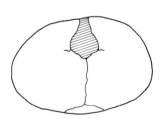

Scaphocephaly
(sagittal suture
synostosis)

Trigonocephaly
(metopic suture
synostosis)

Plagiocephaly
(unilateral coronal
synostosis)

Occipital plagiocephaly
(lambdoid suture
synostosis)

Bilateral coronal
suture synostosis
(as in Apert's and
Crouzon's syndromes)

Craniofacial surgery

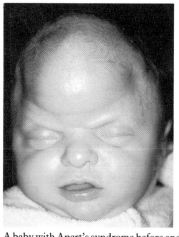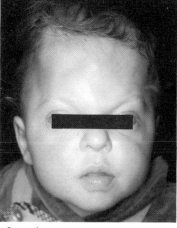

A baby with Apert's syndrome before and after early surgery.

The craniofacial synostoses have in common the premature fusion of the cranial vault sutures together with developmental failure of the growth areas of the skull base and upper face. The deformities that may result are therefore more complex and severe, and surgical correction is more often necessary. Several syndromes fall into this group, the most common being Crouzon's syndrome and Apert's syndrome. Apert's syndrome is sometimes included in a batch of disorders called collectively acrocephalosyndactyly; syndactyly of hands and feet also occurs. These may be genetically transmitted.

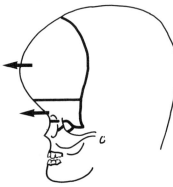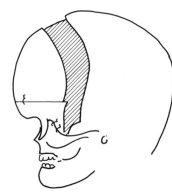

Frontal advancement as carried out for Conzon's and Apert's syndromes showing the bone cuts (——) and open area left free after advancement (▨). The growing brain is then free to push on the forehead.

Surgery in these conditions is directed at relieving raised intracranial pressure and allowing as far as possible for normal growth and development of brain and cranium in infancy. These procedures usually require removal of bone from the sites of the fused sutures in the vault and cranial base where accessible, enlargement of the intracranial volume, and correction of asymmetry in the cranium and upper orbits.

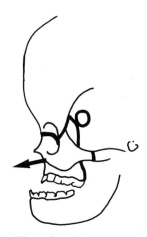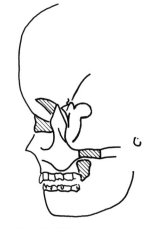

Le Fort III mid-facial advancement showing bone cuts (——) and bone grafts (▨).

Later surgery, generally in early childhood, is directed at correcting any facial deformity, which may be gross. For example in some children with Crouzon's and Apert's syndromes a form of "dish face" develops, with proptosed eyes, resulting from limited growth of the mid-face. This can be vastly improved by a procedure to advance the whole mid-facial skeleton. All this surgery is done as far as possible through an approach via a coronal scalp incision to avoid scars on the facial skin.

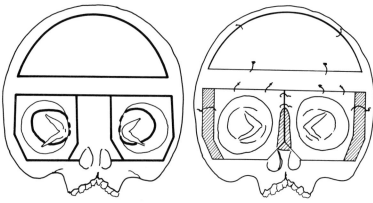

Correction of hypertolerism showing bone cuts (——) and bone grafts (▨).

Orbital problems—The whole of one or both bony orbits may be displaced in any direction as part of a congenital anomaly that may be associated with a facial cleft or zone of hypoplasia, an encephalocoele, or as part of craniofacial synostosis. These abnormalities produce a bizarre facial appearance and, often, visual problems. The commonest anomaly of this type is hypertelorism, in which the orbits are widely separated with an abnormal nose in between. Craniofacial surgical techniques have been developed in which the parts of the orbits containing the eyeballs may be safely moved into more normal relation. This can be done in early childhood. There may be extensive soft tissue deformities in addition to skeletal ones in some of these conditions; these often require further "tidy up" procedures. The ultimate result depends largely on these soft tissue problems and may be short of ideal. Squint surgery is often necessary at some stage in the management of these children.

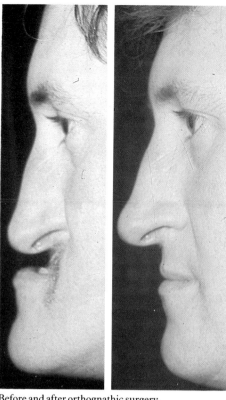

Miscellaneous deformities affecting the head and face are often amenable to surgical correction. Not all of these require combined neurosurgical and plastic surgical procedures, but their management has been made much easier, safer, and more effective as a result of the multidisciplinary approach and new techniques used in craniofacial surgery. Examples of this are the Treacher Collins syndrome and hemifacial microsomia. The Treacher Collins syndrome may be extremely deforming and associated with complex squints as well as problems of dental occlusion. Hemifacial microsomia, with changing facial asymmetry as growth proceeds, similarly has several facets to its management. Many of the children with monstrous abnormalities have, contrary to popular belief, normal intelligence. Consequently, surgical correction to as near normal as possible is worth while and should be done as early as possible. Some patients with these deformities develop abnormalities of jaw relation with consequent effects on facial contour and dental occlusion. These problems are common in patients with clefts of the lip and palate but may be found in others without clefts and are almost always present in those with Apert's and Crouzon's syndromes. Orthognathic surgery as practised by oral and maxillofacial surgeons may thus form part of the multidisciplinary approach and, because of the sensitivity of the mouth to very minor disturbances of dental occlusion, requires careful planning. Complex ancillary technical help is necessary to contribute to positioning and external fixation of the surgical fractures. This work has made an appreciable impact on the management of these patients, with often spectacular improvement in appearance.

Before and after orthognathic surgery.

Tumours and tumour like conditions

Craniofacial tumours and tumour like conditions	
Conditions requiring resection of the cranial base and suited to the craniofacial technique	
Conditions	**Tissue types**
• Inaccessible benign tumours	Skin
• Malignant tumours requiring radical removal	Nasal and paranasal sinus mucosa
	Other epithelial tissues
• Diffuse tumour like conditions (bone dysplasia, neurofibromatosis)	Bones
	Connective tissue

The table shows the tumours that can be dealt with by craniofacial surgical techniques. Patients with tumours in the craniofacial region need careful assessment, with computed tomographic scanning in particular, to define accurately the limits of tumour spread and plan the required resection and reconstruction. Not all tumours in this region require surgery, but it can be used if other methods of treatment are not the most appropriate. The aim in tumours for which surgery is indicated is total removal, and such a resection may include the bone of the skull base if that is affected, the dura mater, and even, if necessary, some of the brain.

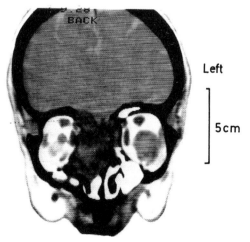

The reconstructive aspects of this surgery are considerable and require repair of the dura, the cranial base, the lining tissues of the nasal roof, and other adjacent structures to produce a well protected cranial cavity and as good an appearance as possible. Success in dealing with craniofacial tumours depends largely on the histological type of growth and on its extent. Appreciable numbers of patients with these until recently inoperable tumours can be salvaged by this surgical approach when carefully selected.

A group of tumour like conditions, which behave like tumours, are also treated by craniofacial resection and repair. The bone dysplasias, which may affect the craniofacial skeleton, in particular fibrous dysplasia, may require surgery. In general, the only way to arrest surgically the progression of the gross bony enlargement that can develop in this condition is to resect (completely if at all possible) the affected area of bone and reconstruct it with bone grafts from unaffected bones. Such procedures are possible. Another tumour like disorder is neurofibromatosis, affecting the region around the orbit, a most difficult condition to treat but one that has been dealt with in craniofacial centres with some degree of success.

Computed tomogram showing a craniofacial tumour, which was successfully resected.

Craniofacial surgery
Craniofacial trauma

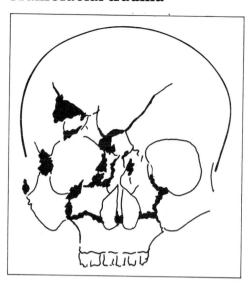

Craniofacial trauma, still a problem despite seat belts, is the third main area where craniofacial surgical techniques have much to offer. Most of this kind of trauma, including extensive damage to the anterior cranial base, frontal sinus, orbits, and jaws, requires a multidisciplinary approach with a neurosurgical, plastic, maxillofacial, and ophthalmic team contributing as necessary to the restoration of satisfactory function and appearance. Generally these cases are managed in regional neurosurgical centres. The combined craniofacial approach has been found to reduce the time in the acute hospital and late complications of trauma. Further surgical procedures—for instance, the reconstruction of traumatically displaced orbits or malunion of the facial bones (difficult technically)—are seldom required.

Craniofacial surgery is an exciting development in reconstructive surgery and has already made startling contributions to the treatment of some of the most difficult and ugly deformities encountered. The future will see refinements of existing surgical techniques and of patient management, probably new applications for this sort of work, and, with further research, a better understanding of the aetiology and the complexities of the congenital craniofacial deformities.

CONGENITAL ABNORMALITIES

Hypospadias

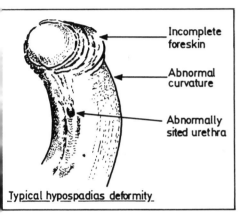

Incomplete foreskin

Abnormal curvature

Abnormally sited urethra

Typical hypospadias deformity

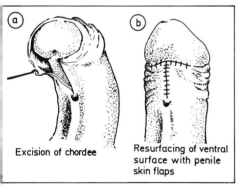

(a) Excision of chordee

(b) Resurfacing of ventral surface with penile skin flaps

Hypospadias is a congenital anatomical disorder of the penis in which the urethral meatus fails to reach the tip of the glans. It occurs in one in every 300 live male births. Subglandular or coronal siting of the urethra is the commonest form, followed by the distal and mid-penile forms and then the much rarer penoscrotal, scrotal, and perineal forms, in which the deformity can be so severe that identification of sex is difficult. The more proximal the urethral orifice the higher is the incidence of associated genitourinary anomalies requiring investigation and treatment.

The anatomical fault is not only of the urethra itself but also of an absent corpus spongiosum between the orifice of the urethra and the base of the glans penis, which is substituted by a fan shaped sheet of fibrous tissue (chordee) to give an abnormal distal curvature that is more obvious on erection. Failure of development of the prepuce on the ventral surface gives a hooded appearance to the penis and exaggerates the ventral curvature. Thus the signs and symptoms of hypospadias are of ventral bowing of the penis and spraying of the urine between the legs, which forces untreated older boys to crouch to pass urine. Chordee is absent or insignificant, however, in the glandular and coronal forms, permitting normal erections and tolerable spraying.

The aim of treatment is to construct in as few operations as possible a penis that looks and functions as normally as possible and has a natural urethral orifice at the tip of the glans, allowing the boy to start primary school without disadvantage. Surgery may not be necessary at all in glandular hypospadias, but, if indicated, the condition deserves a simple meatoplasty as a day case or overnight stay. Coronal hypospadias is treated in one operation, using local flaps to create the new urethra and its covering. More proximal forms of hypospadias commonly require a procedure in two stages: in the first the chordee is meticulously excised before introducing new skin to the defect either as a free, full thickness, prepucial graft or as a prepucial flap that is allowed to "settle" during an interval of six months; in the second a urethroplasty is done.

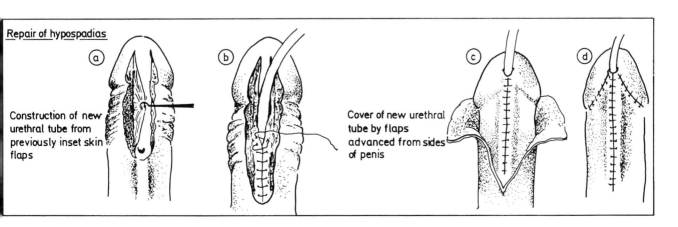

Repair of hypospadias

(a) Construction of new urethral tube from previously inset skin flaps

(b)

(c) Cover of new urethral tube by flaps advanced from sides of penis

(d)

Congenital abnormalities

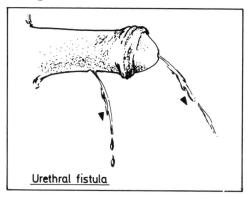

Urethral fistula

At present there is a tendency to attempt repair in one stage, using prepucial and penile flaps, but, regardless of the technique, the child remains in hospital during each operation for not less than 10 days with an indwelling catheter or temporary perineal or suprapubic urinary diversion until the dressings, sutures, and catheters can be removed.

The main complication of repair of hypospadias—namely, penile urethral fistula (incidence seldom less than 10%)—may unfortunately obstruct surgical goals, in which case further surgery to close the fistula is necessary. As residual prepucial skin may be used for repair of the fistula any religious, racial, parental, or professional pressures for formal circumcision must be resisted until a watertight urethra has been constructed to the tip of the penis.

Haemangiomas

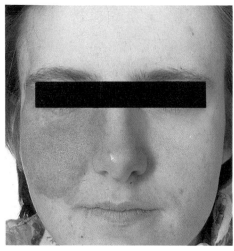

Haemangiomas are the commonest tumours of infancy, occurring in 3% of all neonates and 12% of all 1 year old children. The described varieties have acquired many confusingly impressive eponyms and poetic titles, but essentially the appearance, distribution, and behaviour of a haemangioma depend on the types of vessels it contains, the characteristics of flow within them, and the level at which the vascular complex lies in the skin and subcutaneous tissues.

The portwine stain is a consequence of abnormal intradermal arterial and venous capillaries lying in the facial distribution of one or more of the three sensory branches of the fifth cranial nerve. Apart from the eye catching colour there is a 40% added risk in those patients in whom the ophthalmic and maxillary areas are affected of developing glaucoma or the much rarer complication of intracranial meningeal infiltration by haemangioma in the frontoparietal region with subsequent cerebral symptoms such as epilepsy. Early ophthalmic and neurological assessment and follow up are therefore prudent. Portwine stains tend to darken and, in later adult life, to develop ugly, verrucous lesions. There is no single satisfactory method of treatment, and excision, skin grafting, flap cover, tattooing, superficial diathermy, and even argon laser treatment all have their limitations. The advantages of each method singly or in combination are discussed with the patient and parents before a test patch is treated with the most appropriate technique. More extensive treatment is continued or another method tested according to the later appearances of the area treated. Cosmetics used according to professional advice remain a popular means of camouflaging untreated haemangiomas or the inevitable scars and residual stains that follow surgical treatment but are not well accepted by men.

Treatment advocated for portwine stain

Cosmetic camouflage
Superficial diathermy
Dermabrasion
Argon laser
Serial excision
Excision and graft
Excision and flap

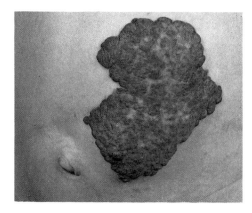

Haemangiomas in the deeper layers of the skin and subcutaneous tissues contain sinusoidal vessels that, depending on their calibre and intra-arterial pressure, take on different sizes and may persist into adult life. They are not always present at birth and may crop up from 2 weeks until 3 months later, growing rapidly to the horror of anxious parents, who must be reassured that nature is the best physician and that, although the haemangioma may continue to increase in size up to 1 year, it will tend to involute spontaneously after that time. Of the more superficial strawberry haemangiomas, 95% will have regressed by the age of six, but about 30% of the deeper cavernous haemangiomas will persist into adult life. Even after involution, however, an unsightly sac of redundant skin may remain, which is easy to tidy up surgically. In the absence of any reliable clinical indices to predict which haemangioma will fail to regress the only indication for early intervention is if breathing, feeding, vision, or voiding are seriously compromised, in which case a short and carefully supervised regimen of treatment with prednisolone is useful; alternatively, surgical excision or, in the last resort, low dose irradiation may be performed. The rare complication of disseminated intravascular coagulopathy (the Kasabach-Merritt syndrome) is best treated medically.

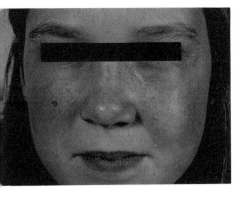

Persistent cavernous haemangiomas in adults are difficult to ablate permanently for, although their bulk and vascularity may be diminished by ligation or superselective therapeutic embolisation of the main arteries before surgical excision, there is a tendency for later revascularisation and recurrence.

Giant pigmented naevus

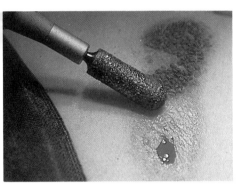

A pigmented naevus is regarded as giant if the defect expected after excision cannot be closed directly and needs a flap or skin graft. It consists of excessive congenital naevus cells within the dermis concentrated particularly around the sebaceous glands and hair bulbs and invading the subcutaneous tissues. The indications for treatment are cosmetic (very reasonably, especially for those on the face, which account for 60% of all giant naevuses) and the potential hazard of malignancy. The true incidence of malignant melanoma in giant naevuses is not known and is quoted as being between 2% and 15%, but whether the risk deserves total excision of very large lesions, such as the bathing trunk naevus, is debatable.

Effective aesthetic treatment is difficult. Neonatal dermabrasion before three months while the naevus cells are lying more superficially in the dermis is appealing, but hairs are not eliminated and patchy pigmentation can recur. Shaving by a skin graft knife has the same limitations, leaving the surgeon with few alternatives to a deeper excision and resurfacing with skin grafts or flaps, with all the concomitant disadvantages of added scarring and donor sites.

Deformities of the ear

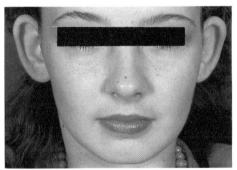

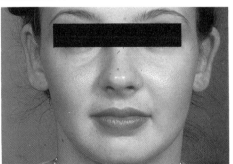

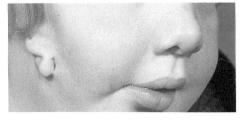

The commonest deformity of the ears is prominent ears secondary to a failure in development of the normal antihelical fold or an abnormally large and deep conchal bowl, or a combination of the two. Parents are naturally concerned on behalf of their baby, especially if they themselves have been teased excessively in childhood for their own "bat" ears. There is no good reason, however, for surgical correction before the age of 6 as the deformity becomes less obvious with growth of the head and early treatment may interfere with normal growth of the ears. Also, children are quite often unaware of the problem and do not suffer at school. It may seem a little unfair that the selection of children for treatment should be based on whether they are appreciably teased, but at least this avoids having to operate, without good reason, on a large number of children.

Treatment is aimed at correcting the anatomical fault through an incision in the back of the ear that becomes a hidden scar as soon as the ear folds back. It is a simple procedure as a day case, using general anaesthesia for younger children and local anaesthesia for older and more resilient children and for adults. Well padded circumferential head bandages are worn for two weeks followed by bandaging at night for a further four weeks.

A rare deformity of the ear is failure in development ranging from anotia to varying degrees of microtia, occasionally associated with middle ear problems, absent external auditory meatus, facial palsy, and craniofacial anomalies. Reconstruction of a convincing, aesthetic ear is difficult and requires a surgical programme in many stages starting from the age of 6 and using a silastic or appropriately carved autogenous cartilage framework implanted within locally mobilised flaps of skin. A compromise sometimes has to be reached whereby attention is paid mainly to constructing the lower third of the ear, leaving the upper part to be obscured by hair grown to the right length. Alternatively, a prosthetic ear can be used that often looks better than one made by several lengthy operations, but this has the disadvantage of being displaced during the normal activities of a growing child.

SKIN COVER

Partial thickness grafts

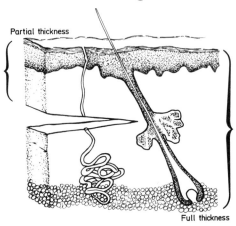

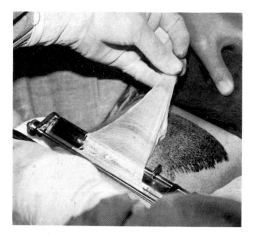

A skin graft is a segment of dermis and epidermis that has been completely separated from its blood supply and is transplanted to another area of the body. The first successful skin graft was performed in France in 1869 by Jacques Reverdan. In this country partial thickness grafts (split thickness or Thiersch's grafts) are harvested as large sheets from either the arm, leg, or buttocks using a blade with an adjustable protective roller at the leading edge, which determines the thickness of the skin. As epidermal remnants are left behind in the donor site the skin heals within 10 to 14 days, depending on the thickness of the graft, usually with only minimal pigment change. If a large area of skin loss needs to be covered the partial thickness graft can be meshed using a machine that permits an expansion in the graft rather like a string vest. Skin grafts can be stored in a domestic fridge if kept moist and used up to three weeks later.

The survival of a skin graft depends on the recipient site being sufficiently vascular to support the metabolic needs of the graft and free from gross infection. A successful "take" also requires immobilisation and the prevention of seromas and haematomas, which may lift the graft off the vascular bed. Gross infection mobilises the fibrinolytic system and breaks down the fibrin adhesion between the graft and the recipient bed. Partial thickness grafts may be applied to a wound directly at the time of surgery and the immobilisation and prevention of seroma obtained by the application of a bolus pressure dressing using proflavine wool or thick foam. Grafts may also be applied 24-28 hours after surgery and left exposed for frequent wound toilet and debridement without any tie-over dressing. The main disadvantages are the cosmetic mismatch between the graft and surrounding normal skin in colour, quality, and contour and the tendency of the wound to contract. So called pinch grafts are not favoured by plastic surgeons principally because of the appalling stippled donor site that is produced in harvesting these grafts.

Full thickness grafts

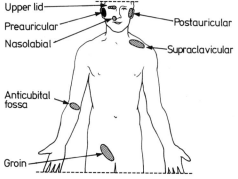

Full thickness (or Wolfe grafts) were first described by a Scottish ophthalmic surgeon John Wolfe, who in 1875 successfully reconstructed a lower eyelid by removing a full thickness graft from the forearm. In this procedure the whole of the epidermis and dermis is transferred; sometimes it may include fat, hair, and sebaceous glands. The advantages of such a graft are the improved cosmetic appearance, the smaller likelihood of contracture, and the possible transfer in certain cases of hair. These grafts are often used for facial reconstruction and can be harvested from behind or in front of the ears, from the upper eyelids or from the supraclavicular region. Similarly, grafts for resurfacing the hand may be harvested from either the groin or the instep of the foot.

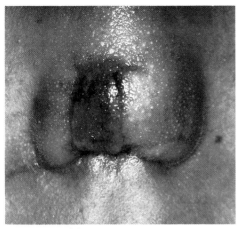
Composite graft from ear.

The disadvantages are that the donor site does not regenerate and therefore has to be primarily closed or itself grafted with a partial thickness skin graft, thus limiting the size of the graft. The recipient bed must possess good vasculature and permit adequate immobilisation; these grafts consequently are often applied using a tie-over bolus dressing.

Skin grafts are initially more susceptible to actinic damage and should therefore be protected for six months. Thin partial thickness skin grafts do not have sebaceous glands and therefore tend to be dry and benefit from the application of lanolin cream. After the initial stage of graft contracture there is a secondary phase of growth in the graft, which parallels the rate of growth of the rest of the body. Scars, however, do not follow this secondary phase, and in children additional surgical procedures may therefore be required where skin grafts have been previously applied, particularly on the hand during adolescence.

Skin flaps

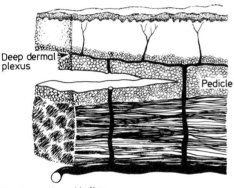
Random pattern skin flap

Skin and its subcutaneous tissue can be moved from one part of the body to another provided the vascular pedicle is maintained between it and the body for nourishment.

Random skin flaps

Most local flaps are raised as random skin flaps and their design is dictated by experience. Their geometric design is only rough, and there are well defined limits to which the length of a flap can be raised despite increasing its width, which limits the safe transfer of skin. The skin in these flaps survives on blood vessels from the subdermal skin plexus, which provides a blood supply many times in excess of the metabolic requirements of the skin. This is because the skin has an important physiological role in regulating temperature. Once raised these flaps may be moved to an adjacent area of skin loss by rotation or transposition.

The design of a random flap obviously presents certain disadvantages in reconstruction. There are two ways of increasing the ratio of length to breadth. Firstly, a flap may be "delayed"; the flap is raised and transferred in more than one stage to ensure its safety. At the first stage a longer flap than would normally survive is incised and partially raised. Ischaemia is thought to be a stimulus to increasing the blood supply to the dermis, possibly by an effect on the capillaries, the delay preventing the shunting of blood away from the dermis. At seven to 10 days a second delay or final raising and transfer of the flap is undertaken. Delaying the skin flap permits roughly a 60-100% increase in survival of flap length. At present despite recent reports flaps cannot be manipulated pharmacologically and the exact physiological basis of delay is not fully understood.

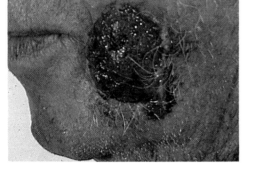
Rotation of random pattern flap.

Secondly, much larger random flaps may be raised by joining two random flaps together, forming a bridge of skin that can be tubed with two pedicles, one at each end. The tube pedicle was introduced in 1916 simultaneously by Sir Harold Gilles in England and Vladimir Filatov, an ophthalmic surgeon, in Russia. At subsequent stages the flap can be divided at one end and inset on to the wrist. At a later stage the other end can be divided, allowing the flap to be transported on the wrist and inset on a distant site on the body. It is, however, a multistage procedure and therefore susceptible to many complications.

Skin cover

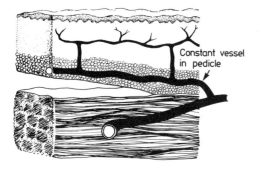

Constant vessel in pedicle

Axial pattern flaps

With the extended use of the previously described random flaps it became evident that on various areas of the body much longer flaps could be raised successfully without delay. McGregor and his colleagues studied such a flap in the groin and were able to raise a flap that was at least four times as long as its base. This was due to there being a constant anatomical blood vessel in the pedicle, in this case the superficial circumflex iliac artery and accompanying veins. It is now known that skin on the anterior chest wall may be raised as a long flap based on perforating branches from the internal mammary artery—the deltopectoral flap. Similarly, the forehead flap, which may be used to resurface areas of the face and oral cavity, is based on the anterior branch of the superficial temporal artery.

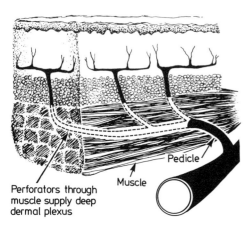

Perforators through muscle supply deep dermal plexus

Muscle

Pedicle

Muscle myocutaneous flaps

Having established the anatomical basis of axial patterned flaps, plastic surgeons searched around the body for similar flaps. It became apparent that large areas of skin were not supplied on an axial basis but were supplied by perforating vessels coming through from underlying muscles. Muscles usually receive their blood supply via a pedicle at one end, and the other end of the muscle may therefore be detached and the muscle isolated on its pedicle with or without the overlying skin. This paddle of muscle can then be rotated through an arc, usually of 360 degrees. If muscle is moved alone skin grafts can be applied to its surface. On the other hand, muscles are often moved with the overlying skin as a myocutaneous flap. The commonly used myocutaneous flaps are pectoralis major used in head and neck reconstruction, latissimus dorsi in breast reconstruction, gluteus maximus in closure of sacral pressure sores, and grastrocnemius in reconstruction around the knee.

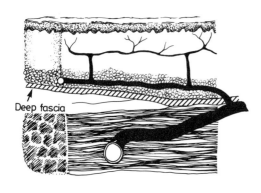

Deep fascia

Fasciocutaneous flaps

More recently it has become evident that there are further areas of skin that are supplied by blood vessels issuing between muscles and supplying a rich vascular plexus that lies just above the deep fascia. This in turn supplies the subdermal plexus of the skin and is the basis of the fasciocutaneous flap that, in certain areas of the body, permits long flaps to be raised for local transposition. Such flaps are important for supplying skin cover to the lower leg and can be raised on the medial or lateral aspects of the shin and transposed over the tibia. Similarly, flaps may be raised from the upper arm or lateral aspect of the thorax for skin cover of the axilla.

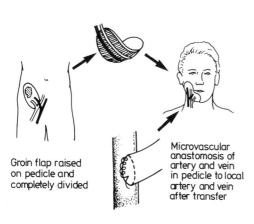

Groin flap raised on pedicle and completely divided

Microvascular anastomosis of artery and vein in pedicle to local artery and vein after transfer

Free flaps

Despite the wealth of flaps that have become available to us there are certain areas of the body that remain extremely difficult to cover, in particular the scalp and the lower leg when there is extensive injury. With the advent of microsurgery, axial pattern flaps, surviving as they do on a single artery and accompanying vein, may be detached from their normal blood supply at the pedicle and the artery and vein anastomosed to a local undamaged artery and vein adjacent to the area of skin loss; provided the anastomoses remain patent these flaps will survive. Muscle and myocutaneous flaps may be similarly transferred as may the more recently described compound flaps such as the deep circumflex iliac artery flap that supplies the skin of the groin, adjacent muscle, and the bone of the iliac crest. This can be moved as a compound flap and used particularly in jaw reconstruction and reconstruction of severe injuries of the tibia.

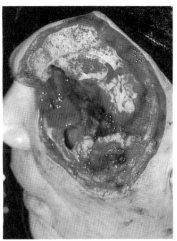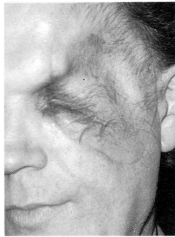

Free scapular flap transfer.

Development of free flaps has permitted the transfer in one stage of tissue to a hostile environment where routine flaps would normally not survive because of the poor vasculature or because of infection. Such procedures, which are now becoming far more routine, although they undoubtedly take more operating time and require the surgical technique of microsurgery, permit a safer and more sophisticated reconstruction than was formerly possible and a greatly reduced stay in hospital compared with the original tube pedicles, which could take at least six months to move into the position in which they were required and had a 50% failure rate.

MICROVASCULAR SURGERY

History		
1902-3	Carrel and Guthrie Hopfner	Successful limb replantation in animals
1963	Che'en *et al* (China)	First successful arm replantation in man
1966	Tamai (Japan)	First successful digit replantation
1969	Cobbett (England)	First toe/thumb transfer
1971	Buncke (USA)	Free omental transfer with revascularisation to cover scalp defect
1972	Harii (Japan)	First successful free flap transfer (scalp)

In 1902 Carrel and Guthrie reported the successful replantation of amputated limbs in dogs using the type of technique in their anastomosis that microvascular surgeons use today. The introduction of the operating microscope by Nylen in 1921 eventually allowed smaller vessels to be successfully repaired, and in 1963 the first successful replantation of an amputated limb was reported in China. In 1966 Tamai was the first surgeon to replant successfully an amputated thumb; this led to the establishment of what has now become a successful and commonplace emergency operation. At the same time the ability to move composite tissues around the body with reanastomosis of their supplying blood vessels to local blood vessels has revolutionised reconstructive surgery since the first successful free flap transfer in 1972.

Replantation

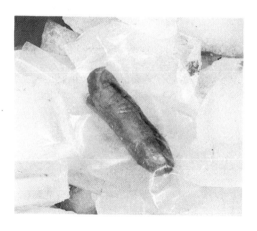

Patients who sustain traumatic amputations of either the whole or part of a limb should be considered for replantation and referred to a centre with particular experience in this work. Before transfer patients must be thoroughly assessed for other less dramatic injuries and if necessary resuscitated with intravenous fluids. In amputation of an arm or leg the period of ischaemia is critical, and several patients have died from renal failure probably produced by the release of free myoglobin. Digits, however, are less susceptible to ischaemia. Amputated members should be placed in a polythene bag, which can then be immersed in iced water before transfer.

Not all amputated members are suitable for replantation, and the selection should be carefully undertaken by an experienced surgeon. A crush or avulsion type injury makes replantation far less satisfactory than does a straight guillotine type injury. The patient's age is important; far better results are obtained in younger patients. A single amputated digit may not always be replanted provided the rest of the hand has full function, but with an amputated thumb replantation is always attempted as its loss represents a 50% reduction in hand function. The table shows other factors taken into consideration.

Criteria for selection
Type of injury
Level of amputation
Number of and the particular digit
Age and coexistent disease
Occupation and patient's wishes
Patient's ability to cooperate with rehabilitation
Length of ischaemia and facilities available

Replantation surgery requires a trained team of surgeons, anaesthetists, and nurses and facilities for prolonged rehabilitation. The operation may be performed under either regional block anaesthesia or general anaesthesia.

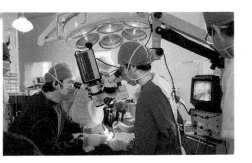

Firstly, the bony skeleton is stabilised and severed tendons repaired. Secondly, blood vessels and nerves are anastomosed and skin cover obtained either by local flaps or skin grafting. Postoperatively the amputated limb requires close monitoring and the vascular anastomosis should be re-explored urgently if any vascular embarrassment occurs. After successful replantation prolonged and intensive rehabilitation is required if the amputated limb is to become of any functional use to the patient, the mere cosmetic survival of an amputated limb no longer being considered to be a success. That these operations are time consuming emergency procedures, expensive in operating time, resources, staff, and, postoperatively, rehabilitation, makes them best suited to centres with suitable resources.

Results of emergency replantation

Arm—the results depend on the nature of the accident, but generally only a fair result is obtained. Cosmetic appearance is usually excellent, but sensation to the hand is only partially recovered. The return in muscle power is poor except at the elbow joint, and in general patients do not return to their original job if it requires two handed coordination.

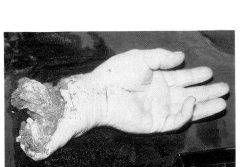

Hand—Much better results are obtained with this amputation, and in 60% of cases reasonable hand function is achieved.

Digit—Seventy five per cent of patients obtain excellent results and are able to resume their original work. They may have a range of motion in the distal joints of 60% of normal, and have a complete or near complete recovery of sensation. The main complications of replantation surgery, particularly of the digits, include intolerance of cold or anaesthesia, or both, and stiffness of adjacent joints. Nerve recovery depends on the extent of the injury but is greatly influenced by the patient's age—that is, younger patients obtain better results than older patients.

Other structures may also be replanted—for example, the scalp, which may be avulsed by long hair being caught in rotating machinery. The lip and nose may be traumatically amputated en bloc and have been replanted successfully, as have amputated ears. Successful replantation of legs has been reported, but function is poor, and even amputated penises have been successfuly replanted. The successful replantation of digits has also permitted the transfer of one or two toes to reconstruct lost thumbs or fingers. Initially the first toe was used, but now more commonly the second toe is transferred. The tissues are moved as a composite unit on the dorsalis pedis artery with accompanying superficial veins together with the digital nerve; these are joined to the appropriate vessels and nerves in the hand. There is minimal functional abnormality in the foot, and the results in the hand from a functional point of view are excellent, particularly in young children.

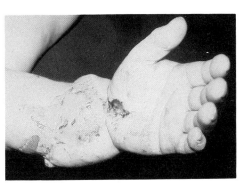

Free flaps

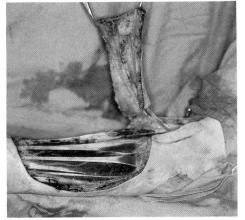

Dissecting radial forearm flap.

The appreciation of the anatomical basis of skin flaps has permitted the successful transfer of skin to distant areas of the body that do not have suitable local flaps. This is achieved by re-establishing their blood supply by anastomosing the artery and vein of their pedicle to a local artery and vein—a so called free flap.

Skin alone may be transferred to reconstruct defects after either a traumatic loss of skin, particularly in the leg, or after excision of tissues for head and neck malignancies. The original flaps used were the groin flap, the deltopectoral flap, and scalp flaps. Skin on the dorsum of the foot based on the dorsalis pedis artery and forearm skin based on the radial artery have more recently been used and have the advantage of permitting the transfer of thin mobile skin, which is of particular advantage in intraoral reconstruction.

In particularly hostile environments, such as follow extensive radiotherapy to the head and neck or chronic osteomyelitis in the leg, free flaps are transferred based on myocutaneous flaps. Such free flaps include the latissimus dorsi and tensor fascia lata muscles. Muscle is thought to be much more capable of withstanding these hostile environments and overcoming radionecrosis or osteomyelitis.

Microvascular surgery

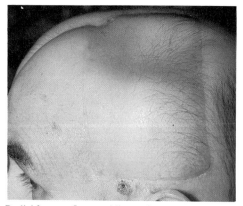

Radial forearm flap providing scalp cover.

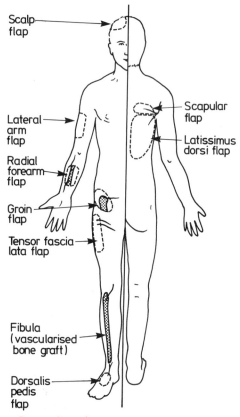

Donor sites of more common free flaps

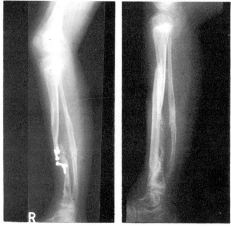

Before and after vascularised fibula graft for
pseudoarthrosis.

The advantages of such free flap techniques are that usually they allow for a one stage operation and in many cases the donor site may be closed primarily or easily hidden from view. The success of such procedures particularly in head and neck reconstruction is at least 90%, comparing very favourably with other types of flaps, particularly with the now almost abandoned tube pedicle.

Because function in many cases is more important than cosmesis both composite flap tissue transfers and specialised tissue transfer have been developed. Composite flaps containing bone, muscle, and overlying skin have been developed for both reconstruction of the jaw and preservation of the leg. The principal ones used are the transfer of iliac crest based on the deep circumflex iliac vessels (the groin flap), the transfer of fibula based on the perineal vessels, and the transfer of part of the radius on the radial forearm flap. Muscle may also be transferred to provide a functional contracting unit, particularly in paralysis of the arm or face. Transfer of muscle obviously requires a successful vascular anastomosis and also reinnervation of the muscle with a local motor nerve. In facial paralysis the operation performed depends on the duration of paralysis. If denervation of the facial muscles has occurred less than one year previously a cross facial nerve anastomosis can be performed using nerve grafts from the sural nerve of the leg as a cable from the facial nerve on the unparalysed side to join with the nerve supplying the paralysed muscle on the affected side. If the paralysis has existed for more than one year these muscles will have wasted and lost their ability to contract. In this case a cross facial nerve graft is combined with a second operation six months later when either the gracilis muscle or pectoralis minor muscle is transferred to the paralysed side of the face and used as motor unit. Its own blood supply is reanastomosed to local blood vessels and its motor nerve joined to the cross facial nerve graft. The quality of the result depends on the nerve anastomoses, but good results have been achieved in younger patients producing bilateral symmetrical facial movement to the lower face.

The microvascular transfer of free tissues has been used on several other organs and structures including joints, nerve, testis, and bowel. In the case of the bowel, after ablative head and neck surgery, large defects in the pharyngeal and cervical oesophagus may be replaced by a segment of jejunum, which can be revascularised by anastomosing its mesenteric vessels to local vessels in the neck. The jejunum is preferred for this procedure because the mesentry is thinner, allowing easier identification of the pedicle compared with the ileum. The colon has also been used in a similar fashion as a conduit either as a free flap or as a pedicle flap and reinforcing its blood supply by anastomosing the marginal artery and vein to vessels in the neck. It does, however, present problems with the discrepancy in size. The transfer of bowel in the way described above is a safe operation with a 90% success rate and has the advantage of being a one stage transfer with an independent blood supply. Its principal disadvantage is that secretions can cause an overspill into the bronchial tree, and in a sick patient laparotomy with bowel anastomosis may have its own complications.

Although microvascular procedures are in many ways still in their infancy and undoubtedly take longer to perform, they have the advantage of being in general one stage procedures. With the use of larger vessels both on the recipient flap and donor site transfers have become far quicker. As a result success rates of up to 90% have been reported, comparing very favourably with other methods of reconstruction. Now that small vessels can be successfully joined together, and once tissue rejection has been solved, composite tissue transfers from cadavers will permit unprecedented possibilities for reconstruction.

Hand replantation courtesy of P Townsend.

BURNS

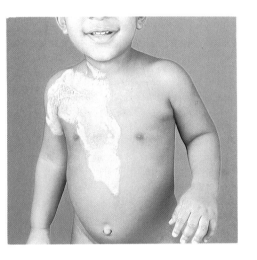

Thermal injury is common, often sustained in the home. Most injuries are minor. Each year, however, 12 000 patients in England and Wales are admitted to hospital, of whom only a small proportion require treatment in a specialised burns unit. The most common injury is that sustained by the inquisitive toddler who pulls down a container of hot liquid over himself, scalding his outstretched arm and often the front of his chest, neck, and face. Burns can produce a heavy workload for a hospital and considerable morbidity for the patient. Their management requires an understanding of not only the pathophysiology of the local skin injury but also the vascular, metabolic, immunological, and psychological changes.

Pathophysiology

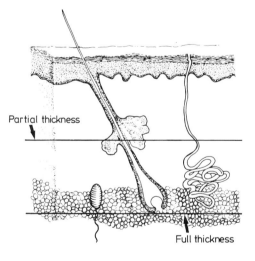

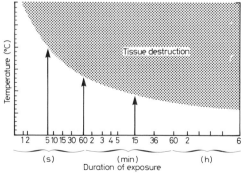

Burns may be classified as partial thickness (will heal spontaneously from epithelial remnants that survive deep in the dermis provided that these are not killed by dehydration or infection) or full thickness (all epithelial appendages are destroyed and epithelialisation therefore can occur only slowly from the edges of the wound; a skin graft will generally be required to achieve skin cover).

The depth of tissue destruction is a function of the temperature and duration of exposure. Most burns do not require enormous temperatures, and tissue destruction can occur at only 45°C provided this is applied for long enough.

Within a major burn injury will not be uniformly deep. Centrally there is a zone of coagulation where cells are irreversibly damaged. Surrounding this is a zone of stasis in which, although the cells are injured, they can survive if the burn is correctly treated. Outside this is a zone of hyperaemia in which the cells are minimally injured and will recover within seven days.

The stratum corneum (the superficial layer of the epidermis) has been described as the waterproof mackintosh of the body. When it is destroyed, as in both deep and superficial burns, water will be lost from the body by evaporation. At the same time the underlying capillaries of the dermal plexus will dilate and fluid and large protein molecules will be lost into the surrounding extracellular space. This will become apparent as oedema and blisters. In addition, in larger burns systemic changes will occur, affecting the heart and lungs and other undamaged tissues, which will also tend to take up water. This fluid loss, which is greatest in the first few hours and continues for at least 36 hours, will if large enough lead to the clinical state of shock. For this reason patients require resuscitation with intravenous fluids. The fluid loss is not greatly influenced by the depth of the injury.

Burns
Management

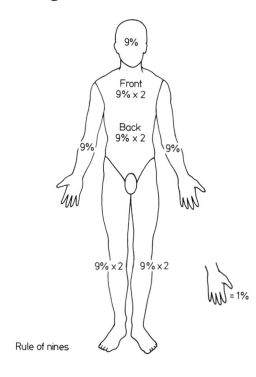

Rule of nines

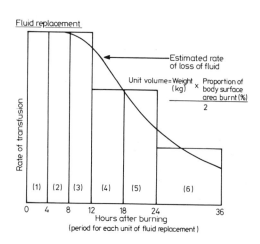

Treatment of major burns

Check airway / vital signs

Assess injury

Set up reliable intravenous drip

Take blood to assess blood group for
cross match, haemoglobin, and packed cell volume

Give analgesics and tetanus toxoid
(steroids if respiratory burn suspected)

Catheterise bladder

Estimate size of burn

Weigh patient

Calculate necessary plasma replacement

Attend to burn wound

Reassess fluid requirement and look out for
complications

History

Important factors are:

The patient's age—burns at the extremes of age (less than 3 years and greater than 60) have a greater morbidity and mortality.

The type of injury—electrical burns tend to be deeper than scalds.

The time of the accident—fluid replacement should be calculated from this time not from when the patient entered the casualty department.

Other relevant medical conditions—for example, alcoholism, epilepsy, diabetes, artherosclerosis, drug abuse.

Examination

Size—This may be expressed as a proportion of the total body surface area, which may be easily assessed by the "rule of nines," noting also that the palm of the hand is equivalent to 1% of the body surface area. Different calculations are required for children because the head is larger relative to the rest of the body. In general, burns greater than 10% in children or 15% in adults will necessitate intravenous fluid replacement. Smaller burns can be managed by oral fluid replacement.

Depth—The depth of a burn may be difficult to diagnose initially, especially in children. In general, if the burnt area is erythematous in colour and blanches on pressure it is of partial thickness. Similarly, if the burnt area retains pin prick sensation (repeated light pricking over a small area) the injury is probably of partial thickness as the nerve endings tend to lie just below the deepest penetration of the sweat glands—that is, at the lowest level of epithelial cells.

Location—Burns of the face, neck, hands, feet, and perineum may cause special problems and warrant careful attention.

Treatment

The table gives the 11 most important steps in treatment of major burns.

First aid treatment—Remove overlying clothing immediately as heat is retained within the fibres of the garment. Then immerse the damaged area in cold water for at least 10 minutes and preferably much longer. This immediately cools the damaged skin and underlying structures and will prevent further damage.

Fluid replacement—For larger burns intravenous fluid replacement is required to prevent the development of the clinical state of shock. The amount of fluid will depend on the size of the burn and the size of the patient. More fluid is lost in the first 12 hours but it continues to be lost for at least 36 hours. No general agreement has been reached on the best type of fluid for resuscitation. At least five different types are recommended but all have one thing in common: they contain sodium and water. The amount of fluid infused should effectively provide 0·5-0·6 mmol(mEq) sodium and 2-4 ml water/kg body weight/% body surface area damaged. In the United Kingdom plasma protein fraction is the most commonly used replacement fluid. It is usually administered according to a formula devised by Muir and Barcley, which provides an initial guide to the amount of fluid to be given. The initial resuscitation period of 36 hours is divided into six unequal periods, in each of which an equal volume of plasma is given. This volume of plasma is calculated by multiplying the percentage surface area of the burn by the weight (kg) of the patient and dividing by two. This figure gives the volume (ml) that should be infused. At the end of the first four hour period the patient is assessed, and if fluid replacement is adequate as judged by mental state, pulse rate, blood pressure, quality and quantity of urine output, blood haemoglobin concentration, and proportional cell volume it is repeated again for a further period.

Additional fluids are required to replace the normal, daily metabolic requirements of roughly 3 l crystalloid fluid for an adult. In larger, deeper burns destruction of red blood cells also occurs, which may require blood transfusion in the second 24 hours of resuscitation.

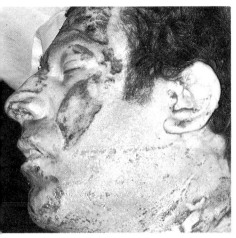

External evidence of a respiratory burn.

Inhalation injury

The inhalation of poisonous gases is the single most lethal component of a burn and should always be looked for at the initial assessment. Apart from the history of the accident having occurred in an enclosed space, examination may show burnt skin around the mouth and nostrils with carbon inside the nose and oedema of the oral, nasal, and pharyngeal mucosa. Inhaled hot air damages the upper respiratory tract and, in particular, produces oedema of the larynx. This is usually diagnosed early and can be compounded by hypoxia, the inhalation of carbon monoxide and, particularly in a domestic setting, very toxic gases such as hydrogen cyanide, which are released from the combustion of synthetic modern upholstery. The damage produced by these chemicals tends to become apparent later and affect the lower respiratory tract leading to atelectasis and pneumonia. Investigations include baseline chest radiography, monitoring of blood gas and serum carbon monoxide concentrations, and examination of the upper respiratory tract by laryngoscopy and fibreoptic bronchoscopy. Treatment rests on the inhalation of humidified air, correction of pulmonary oedema, and the administration of prophylactic antibiotics. Treatment with a short course of high dose steroids may be helpful. More severe injuries require oxygen treatment, and if the blood gases deteriorate positive pressure ventilation may be required. Tracheostomies are generally best avoided.

Important factors in electrical injury

- Type of current
- Voltage of current
- Amperage of current
- Resistance offered by body
- Pathway of current through body
- Duration of contact

Complications of electrical injury

- Cardiac arrest
- Renal failure
- Renal calculus
- Spinal cord damage
- Cataract formation

Electrical injury

Resistance to the flow of electrical current results in the production of heat. Bone has the highest resistance, followed by in descending order, fat, muscle, skin, blood vessels, and, least of all, nerves. Skin epidermis is non-vascular and offers a high resistance when dry, but this resistance is proportional to the thickness of the skin, its temperature, and the amount of moisture it contains. Skin can be damaged by either the flow of electricity through it, an arcing injury, or by the ignition of clothing causing flame burns. Deeper damage depends on the path of the electric current. Passage along bone produces the greatest heat and will result in adjacent deep muscle damage. The indication for a fasciotomy (releasing of the deep fascia) may not initially be evident. Delay results in even more muscle necrosis from ischaemia caused by the unrelieved oedema. The passage of the current along blood vessels can produce intimal damage with vessel thrombosis. This will in turn produce tissue death, which may become apparent only later. Both these factors account for many electrical burns being far more extensive than was apparent at the initial examination.

Agents causing chemical burns			
Agent	Common use	Cleansing and dilution	Special treatment
Lime	Agriculture Cement	Brush off, then water	
Oxidising agents			
Potassium permanganate Sodium hypochlorite	Disinfectants, bleach, deodorisers	Water	
Chromic acid	Metal cleansing	Water	
Corrosives phenols			
Phenols	Deodorisers, sanitisers, disinfectants	Ethyl alcohol	
White phosphorus	Armaments industry	Water and debride particles	Irrigate with 1% $CuSO_4$
Hydrofluoric acid	Etching	Water	Topical calcium cream

Chemical burns

The severity of a chemical burn depends on the agent encountered, its concentration and quantity, and the length of time the tissues are in contact with it. Chemical burns are often deeper than they initially appear to be and may progress with time. Initial treatment is dilution of the chemical, which is usually best achieved by prolonged submersion in continuous running water. In general, neutralising agents are contraindicated as they may cause exothermic reactions and increase tissue damage. Damage to the eye should be managed by initial copious irrigation with saline or water, and an ophthalmic opinion should be obtained.

Burns

Management of the burn wound

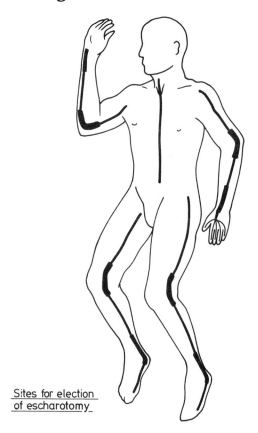

Sites for election of escharotomy

Treatment is initially aimed at relieving pain, which is greatest in superficial burns. This is best achieved by covering the exposed injury with a dressing, which should also provide optimum conditions for epithelial regeneration. Dehydration and infection are the two principal causes of epithelial death, and the dressing should be designed to prevent these occurring. Prophylactic antibiotics are not generally given, but topical antiseptic agents are often used, for example, silver sulphadiazine cream, which is particularly effective, against pseudomonas. In children the depth of the burn is difficult to diagnose; consequently, most are treated initially by conservative measures and spontaneous healing awaited for two to three weeks. Any area that has not healed after this time may be regarded as full thickness and treated with skin grafting. In specialist hands there is a case for early excision and grafting for this type of injury. Adults with an obvious well circumscribed full thickness burn are best treated by early excision and grafting before infection develops. Larger burns treated in specialised units are usually serially excised and skin grafted as donor site skin becomes available.

Deep circumferential burns require special consideration. In the arms and legs they can embarrass the circulation and about the thorax they can restrict respiratory movements. The eschar in these cases should be divided longitudinally, which can be done without any form of anaesthesia. Eyelid damage presents a serious threat if the cornea is exposed. Fortunately, full thickness damage is rare, and split thickness skin grafts applied under Stent moulds permit resurfacing of the lids.

Dressings

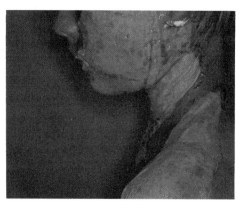

Lyophilised pig skin.

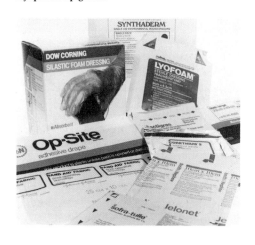

The standard burn dressing consists of gauze impregnated with soft paraffin, which helps to prevent adherence to the wound. A topical antiseptic may be applied over this followed by cotton wool or Gamgee to absorb the exudate. Newer dressings have been introduced that are claimed to be less adherent and allow less water to be lost by evaporation from the wound while also protecting it from external pathogens. These may be classified into two groups:

(1) *Biological dressings*—These may be of homograft or heterograft skin—for example, porcine or amnion. They can be used either fresh or after storage following preparation by freezing in liquid nitrogen or rapid dehydration (lyophilisation) and later reconstitution with saline. One of the more commonly used is lyophilised pig skin. Pig skin was originally used as a dressing in the late 1800s but it had to be abandoned because of antivivisection pressure at that time. It was reintroduced in 1965. Whichever dressing is used, it principally consists of an adherent collagenous dermal surface and a keratinised waterproof epidermis. Criticisms of these dressings go back 130 years to Dupuytren, who described "incorporation into the integument," and antibodies may be shown as a response to foreign proteins trapped within the dermis.

(2) *Physiological dressings*—These consist of synthetic materials such as polyethylene or silicone, which prevent adherence to the wound, and plastic films, which reduce evaporation and contamination.

Late treatment

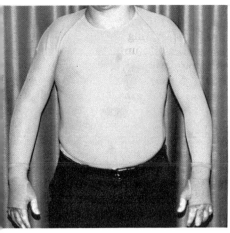

Pressure garment.

On discharge from hospital patients will require regular review. Treatment is directed at relieving the initial local symptoms, which are usually quite severe itching and dryness. Lanolin (face cream) can be lightly massaged into the grafted area. Topical pressure as provided by elasticated, individually made garments has radically altered the management of these patients. Not only does it alleviate the itching symptoms but it has also been shown to prevent contractures. Scarring can impose severe functional and cosmetic disability. Where there is functional limitation of movement at joints or around the orifices of the face release of the scars with skin grafting is required. Many patients, however, are referred later with cosmetic deformities. Shaving of the wounds down so that they are flat followed by overgrafting has not proved a satisfactory way of managing these patients, and some may therefore require prolonged psychological support.

SCARS, HYPERTROPHIC SCARS, AND KELOIDS

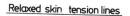
Relaxed skin tension lines

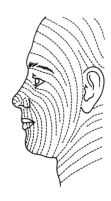

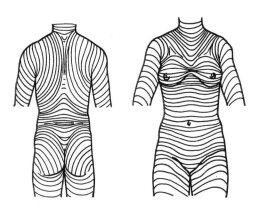

Plastic surgeons have the enviable reputation with the lay public of being able to produce invisible scars, but unfortunately this goal cannot be attained. All surgeons try to produce a slender, pale scar that is flat, but despite great attention to surgical technique some patients develop an itchy raised, and broad scar that is unattractive. Several factors influence the final cosmetic appearance of a scar:

The site on the patient—Scars tend to be excellent on the eyelids but poor on the shoulders and presternal regions. Elective incisions should be placed so that the underlying muscles apply the least tension across the wound. These are not consistent with Langer's lines or, always, with the skin creases of old age, though the second are a good guide. The relaxed skin tension lines may be derived by pinching the skin and observing the ease and size of the furrows and ridges formed. Pinching at right angles to the relaxed skin tension lines is performed with greater ease and produces a longer furrow, and it is along this line that the scar should be placed. Collagen in the dermis is predominantly orientated in a plane perpendicular to the underlying muscle pull. The collagen formed in scars is parallel to the long axis of the scar. Thus a scar placed perpendicular to the muscle pull will heal with collagen fibres orientated in the same direction as normally present. The scar will then merely be an accentuation of the normal pattern.

The age of the patient—Old people tend to develop almost invisible scars on the face, whereas younger patients tend to develop livid scars. Interestingly, pregnant women develop scars that behave like those in children.

The amount of pigmentation—Dark skinned people are far more likely than lighter skinned people to develop a keloid.

A family history of keloid formation may be important, but this has not been statistically proved.

The shape of the scar—A U or V shaped scar tends to form a raised trap door because of poor lymphatic drainage and unequal scar contraction, especially if the injury is shelving.

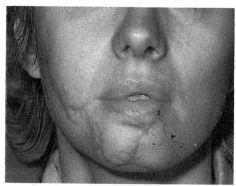
Trap door scar.

Pathophysiology of wound healing

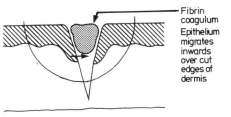

Fibrin coagulum
Epithelium migrates inwards over cut edges of dermis

Five to eight days

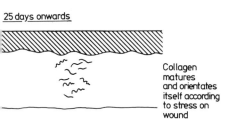

Epithelium migrates along suture and begins to fill wound space

Fibroblasts appear and lay down collagen

25 days onwards

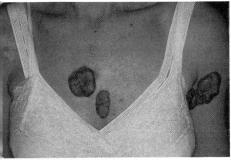

Collagen matures and orientates itself according to stress on wound

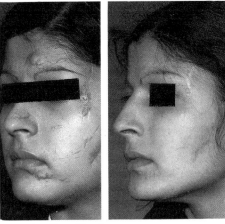

Keloid scars.

The edges of a surgically incised wound are neatly opposed with a suture and the wound edges carefully everted. Histological examination of the healing wound shows many complex cellular reactions. The surface of the wound becomes covered with a fibrin coagulum that seals off the edges of the wound. The epithelial wound edge almost always becomes inverted, grows down into the wound over the dermis to the level of the dermal fat junction, and within five days has migrated across and underneath the fibrin plug. At one week there is a solid core of epithelium in the wound that communicates with a spur of epithelium that has grown down every skin suture track. At about two weeks there is regression of the invasive spur down in the wound and also of the epithelium lining the suture track. At a deeper level in the dermis healing occurs by the invasion of blood capillaries and fibroblasts, the fibroblasts laying down initially immature collagen. This is followed by a much longer phase of scar maturation. This lasts for many months, in which the collagen content increases slowly but mainly undergoes maturation and remodelling so that the collagen bundles reorientate themselves in the scar depending on local forces. At the same time some fibroblasts mature into myofibroblasts, which have the ability to contract and produce scar contracture.

Stress is important as it not only influences the arrangement of the collagen fibres but also determines the activity of the myofibroblasts. Scar contractures tend to occur over the flexor surfaces of joints but not so readily on the extensor aspect. This is partly in response to compression and buckling forces, which stimulate the formation of more collagen, and the contraction of the myofibroblasts, resulting in thick, hypertrophic scars on the flexor aspects of joints.

Clinically, a healed scar initially goes through a red, raised period. Over six months to one year this matures to produce a hypopigmented, flat scar. In some patients, for no particular reason other than the factors mentioned above, the scar goes on to become increasingly red, raised, and itchy. The scar at this point is described as being hypertrophic. If after a year it continues with these symptoms and also tends to invade the surrounding, unaffected, normal tissue as well as increasing in height it is called a keloid scar (derived from the Greek word kelis meaning claw like). The exact clinical differentiation between a hypertrophic scar and a keloid scar is not distinct, and there is no histological difference between the two, but if such scars are compared with a normal scar considerable increases are seen in the amount of immature collagen present. Interestingly, only man forms keloids.

Management of scars

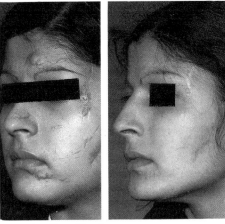

Scar maturation without surgery.

Traumatic scars

The most important time to influence the cosmetic result of a scar is at the time of its initial repair. In traumatically induced lacerations thorough debridement of anaesthetised wounds is required together with a conversion of ragged injuries into straight edged wounds and sutured using an atraumatic technique. In general, interrupted cutaneous sutures should be left in situ for only a few days to avoid cross hatching marks. I advocate the use of a subcuticular suture in most positions on the body except the face. In general, once initial repair of the wound has been undertaken the scar should be left alone to mature for up to one year. This is because many scars that start out red and appear cosmetically unattractive will with maturity fade and become less obvious. A scar should be excised early only if it will obviously require revision at a later date, either because it contains foreign material producing tattooing or because it is distorting anatomical features.

In general the late revision of scars can only produce improvements in the contour by correcting the contour or anatomical distortion. Stretched flat scars are not always helped and in general the line of the scar needs to be altered in these cases by incorporating a z plasty. This, however, results in extra scarring being produced.

Scars, hypertrophic scars, and keloids

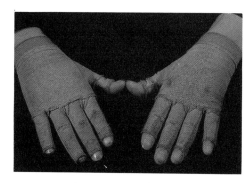

Intralesional steroid injection.

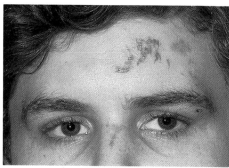

Hypertrophic and keloid scars

Hypertrophic and keloid scars are extremely difficult to treat satisfactorily. When presented with a scar and an intradermal tumour of unknown aetiology, the diagnosis of a keloid should always be borne in mind as simple excision may result in a larger and more unsightly scar being produced. The following therapeutic measures may, however, help:

Intralesional steroids—Triamcinolone may be injected intralesionally or applied topically as a cream. This will in most cases cure itching and in some cases improve the pigmentation. Its disadvantage is that if overused it will produce a hypotrophic, depigmented, thin scar with telangectasia, which may be equally unattractive.

Intralesional excision—Excision within the borders of the keloid tumour produces variable results.

Surgical excision with perioperative or postoperative superficial *x* ray treatment of 16 Gy (1600 rad) in four fractions, the first preferably being given immediately before operation, can give good results in difficult keloids. I appreciate that some clinicians believe that superficial *x* ray treatment is never indicated for a benign condition and certainly would not advocate its use in very young patients or on the lower abdomen in women of childbearing age. I would reserve it for cosmetically disfiguring cases of the head and neck.

Topical pressure hastens collagen maturation and flattens the scar. Treatment should be started early and requires an individually measured elasticated garment to be made. It should be worn both day and night for at least one year or until the symptoms have improved permanently. In general, the garments are well tolerated except on the head and neck and they are the favoured treatment for extensive scarring after burns. Topical pressure has the particular advantage over the two previously described treatments of not having any particular complications, except in children, in whom pressure garments on the thorax have in a few cases interfered with growth of the spine, causing a scoliosis.

Tattoos

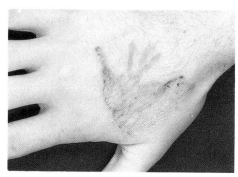

Traumatic tattoo.

Tattoos may be either traumatic or acquired deliberately as part of body adornment. The former occur after explosions or lacerations in which a pigmented foreign material impregnates the wound and is not debrided at the initial time of injury. Most contaminated wounds can be cleaned by scrubbing with a stiff brush, but if the foreign bodies are deeper they should be picked out individually with a hypodermic needle or each wound should be laboriously excised. Wounds that have healed and are tattooed by a foreign body require excision.

Decorative tattoos may be either self induced, usually with a pin and indian ink, or professionally obtained. The standard treatment is the same for both. The tattoo is shaved down in layers with a skin grafting knife, either under local or general anaesthetic, until all the pigment has been removed. In most cases the pigment lies below the dermis and a skin graft is required for the wound to heal.

In recent years lasers have been introduced into clinical practice. There were several optimistic reports on the results of the use of carbon dioxide lasers, but this energy beam not only evaporates the ink pigment but also destroys the overlying skin. Thus it necessarily produces scarring and is indicated only in small amateur tattoos. The argon laser has also been advocated for removing tattoos, and some good results may be obtained with small indian ink tattoos. In general, however, results are disappointing and not invisible, and the process is extremely tedious for the operator to perform. A law has recently been introduced to limit the use of lasers to establishments that are licensed.

Result of laser excision of tattoo.

BENIGN SKIN TUMOURS AND CONDITIONS

The skin is the largest organ of the body. In the average adult it weighs 4 kg and has a volume of 3·6 l and a surface area of 1·8 m². Its many functions include protection against fluid loss by evaporation, regulation of body temperature, and the production and storage of vitamins D and C. It is also a principal organ of sensation. It is a complex structure, composed of the dermis covered by epidermis, the former including many elements such as collagen, elastin, muscle, nerve endings, blood vessels, and fat as well as sweat glands and hair follicles. No wonder, therefore, cutaneous lesions are both common and varied in their pathology. Most patients consult a clinician either for reassurance that a lesion is not malignant or on cosmetic grounds. Although no specific treatment is required, lesions may need to be removed for histological confirmation of the clinical diagnosis. Here I review various types of benign skin lesions and their treatments; they have been selected because of their commonness or importance in plastic surgery.

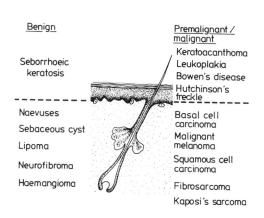

Benign

Seborrhoeic keratosis

Naevuses
Sebaceous cyst
Lipoma
Neurofibroma
Haemangioma

Premalignant / malignant

Keratoacanthoma
Leukoplakia
Bowen's disease
Hutchinson's freckle

Basal cell carcinoma
Malignant melanoma
Squamous cell carcinoma
Fibrosarcoma
Kaposi's sarcoma

Naevus

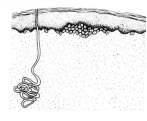

Proliferation of normally situated melanocytes produces a junctional naevus

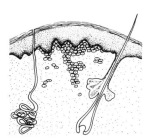

Regression of junctional activity results in an intradermal naevus

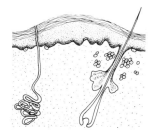

Invasion of dermis produces a compound naevus

A naevus is a tumour of cells that are DOPA positive—that is, can convert dihydroxyphenylalanine into melanin. Usually the melanin is situated in melanocytes in the basal layer of the epidermis. Some authorities consider these cells to be ectodermal, while others think that they are derived from neural elements—that is, from neuroectoderm that migrates into the epidermis. Types of naevus include:

Intradermal naevus—This may be flat or raised, brown or black, with or without hair. The naevus cells are usually confined to the dermis.

Junctional naevus—This is a smooth, flat, pigmented lesion, which may occur on any part of the body, usually in childhood or adolescence. It is particularly common on transitional epithelium such as the vermilion of the lip. There is an appreciable proliferation of naevus cells at the junction of the dermis and epidermis.

Compound naevus—This possesses the features of both a junctional and an intradermal naevus.

Blue naevus—This is a well defined, small intradermal nodule of dermal melanocytes situated deep in the dermis.

Giant pigmented naevus—This occurs most often on the trunk and is characterised by large, darkly pigmented, hairy patches. The skin may be thickened and varucous. It has a tendency to follow a dermatome distribution, is present at birth, and may continue to grow for several years. Such a naevus may undergo malignant change, an incidence of up to 15% being reported by various authors. About 40% of all childhood malignant melanomas, which are extremely rare, occur in these lesions.

Benign skin tumours and conditions

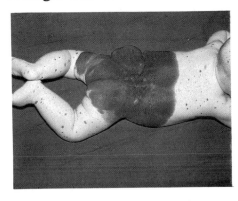

Seborrhoeic keratoses

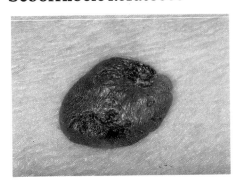

Fibrous tumours

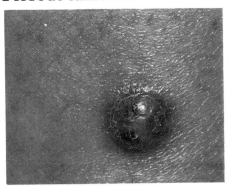

Excision of a cutaneous lesion

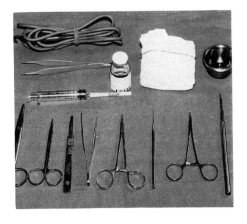

Management

None of these naevuses are in themselves premalignant and most are excised for either functional or cosmetic reasons. Any cutaneous lesion that undergoes change, be it in size, colour, itching, or elevation, should, however, be excised for histological examination.

One treatment of the giant pigmented naevus is complete removal with skin grafting, but some surgeons are now reverting to more conservative management.

Sharing giant naevuses within the first three months of life can produce a considerable cosmetic improvement but has no effect on hair growth. This is because the melanocytes at this time lie more superficially in the epidermis.

Seborrhoeic keratoses vary in size up to 4 cm in diameter. They are usually raised and brown. Characteristically they appear as if stuck on to the skin. The surface of the lesion may appear to have comidome plugs and may be soft and greasy (sebum—tallow, rhoea—flow). These lesions become increasingly apparent with advancing age, even though they may have a congenital aetiology, being dominantly inherited. They are benign tumours of epidermal cell origin. Clinically they are important because if they present atypically they may be confused with either malignant melanoma or squamous cell carcinoma. They can be removed by shaving down rather than by primary excision.

Cutaneous tags and papillomas occur in various sizes and are sessile or pedunculated. They often occur with seborrhoeic keratosis and more often in women than men. They increase in number when the subject gains weight. These lesions are easily removed by excision or electrocautery. Dermatofibroma is a common benign lesion that is firm to palpation and varies from red or brown to yellow. They occur most often on the legs and feet but may also appear on the arms and trunk. They rarely exceed 1·5 cm in size and consist of fibroblasts and collagen. Aetiologically they may be related to minor injury. The histiocytoma is a similar lesion consisting of histiocytes phagocytosing fat rather than fibroblasts producing collagen.

Minor surgery should be practised under conditions that are comfortable for both the patient and the operator. The instruments used should be appropriate to the operation, not a monument to the development of surgical instruments. The lesion should be anaesthetised with a local anaesthetic and a bloodless field provided by incorporating a solution of adrenaline, provided that there is no medical or anatomical contraindication for this (for example, 1% lignocaine with 1/200 000 adrenaline). Five minutes should elapse between infiltration and incision to allow the adrenaline to work. Most lesions are best excised as an ellipse, which should be marked out primarily with a surgical pen. The skin should be stretched in two directions, the best way of doing this without an assistant being to place the handle of the scissors over the lesion. A good working principle is that all lesions should be sent for histological examination. The wound may be sutured in two layers, the subcutaneous tissue being closed with an absorbable suture on an atraumatic cutting needle. The skin should be sutured with an appropriate suture, again on an atraumatic cutting needle. Sutures on the face should not be left in for more than five days. Small lesions on the trunk, arms, and legs may be excised "in the round" and left to heal without any suture. A small depressed scar is left, which is often cosmetically superior to the flat but stretched scar resulting from an elliptical excision.

Cysts

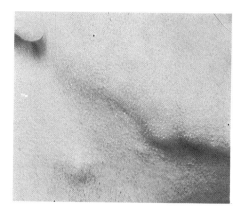

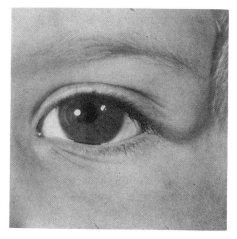

The term "sebaceous cyst" should no longer be used as in most cases sebaceous cells play no part in the formation of these cysts.

Epidermal cysts—These (synonymous with sebaceous cysts) are slow growing intradermal or subcutaneous lesions usually presenting in the face and neck; they may occasionally form part of Gardner's syndrome. They are attached to the overlying normal skin by the remains of the expanded gland duct, showing on the surface as a punctum. Histologically the wall of the cyst is composed of epidermis, but as it matures the wall becomes thinner and the cells flattened.

Pilar cysts, or wens, are clinically similar to epidermal cysts but occur on the scalp. They originate from the middle part of the hair follicle epithelium, and their contents (keratin, fat, and cholesterol) are odourless as they do not become rancid. Simple excision is the treatment of choice; the doctor should ensure that the lining of the sac is completely removed or recurrence is likely. Infected cysts are best treated with antibiotics and excised when quiescent. Occasionally, infected cysts may require drainage. Milia or white heads are tiny (1-2 mm), superficially situated epidermal inclusion cysts. They tend to occur around the eyes in particular, where they may be confused with xanthelasma, and also occur on dermabrasion sites. Treatment is by simple excision or carbon dioxide laser.

Dermoid cysts are subcutaneous lesions usually presenting at birth and often situated on the face around the eyes. They result from sequestration of the skin along the lines of embryonic closure. They may be adherent to periosteum and often develop deep extensions. The cyst is lined by epidermis but may contain various epidermal appendages such as hair follicles. Surgical excision may develop into a "tour de force," and complete excision may require wide exposure of structures around the orbit and nose. They are best referred for specialist opinion.

Inclusion dermoid cysts (epidermal inclusion cysts) result from the traumatic implantation of a fragment of skin into the subcutaneous tissues. A cystic swelling, lined by squamous epithelium containing cholesterol and keratin, results. They are common on the palmar aspect of the hand as a result of minor trauma.

Neurofibromatosis

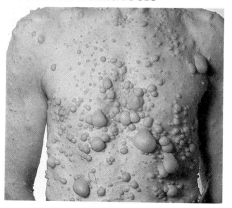

Von Recklinhausen's neurofibromatosis is a hereditary disorder that presents with multiple cutaneous neurofibromas and café au lait pigmentation of the skin. The patient may also have neurofibromas throughout the rest of the body resulting in, for example, bone lesions or gastrointestinal symptoms. Although the skin pigmentation may have been present since birth or early childhood, tumour formation is generally most aggressive at the time of puberty. The disease is unpredictable, but there is a rough correlation between the age at onset of the neurofibromas and the severity of the disease. Treatment consists of excising lesions, giving rise to symptoms because excising all the lesions is usually impossible. Very occasionally malignant degeneration may occur.

Rhinophyma

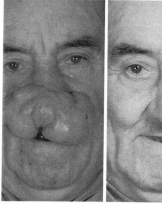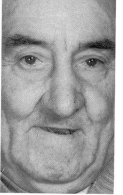

Rhinophyma is a clinical presentation of acne rosacea. The sebaceous glands of the skin are increased in size by the ducts being dilated and filled with keratin. This produces the characteristic enlargement and disfigurement of the nose. The condition has nothing to do with drinking too much alcohol. Treatment on cosmetic grounds is simply to shave the lesion down using a large scalpel blade until a nose of normal size and shape is obtained. The epithelium regenerates spontaneously from the epithelial remnants that are left behind. This procedure may be done under local anaesthetic.

Benign skin tumours and conditions
Hyperhydrosis

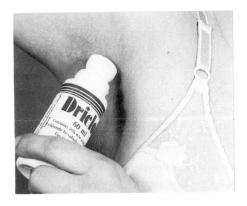

Excessive sweating may be either generalised all over the body or limited to one particular area. It is a condition often affecting the axilla, producing gross discomfort and social embarrassment. After ruling out any serious systemic disturbance the first line of treatment is the topical application of aluminium chloride in an alcoholic solution (aluminium chloride hexohydrate in 20% alcoholic solution). The solution is applied to the dry axilla before going to bed and washed off the next morning. The site of application must be dry if local irritation is to be avoided. The frequency of treatment is reduced as the condition improves. It is not known how this solution works, but possibly it causes protein precipitation that blocks the sweat duct orifices. If a local hypersensitivity reaction occurs it may be helped by 0.5% hydrocortisone cream; the reaction may, however, be severe enough to necessitate stopping the treatment. Only those patients in whom a prolonged course of medical treatment fails or who have severe hypersensitivity reactions are referred for surgical treatment. If the process affects the axillas and the hands the patient may be better served by cervical sympathectomy. This is, however, a major operation, and the symptoms may return after a year or two. If, however, the condition is localised to the axillas excision of an ellipse of skin containing the major part of the sweat glands is the treatment of choice. This may be done as a day case procedure. Various refinements on this procedure have been introduced because scars in the axilla may cause appreciable trouble. In particular, they may result in a limitation of abduction and extend on to the anterior axillary fold and thus be visible. In one alternative procedure the subcutaneous tissues are cleared by curetting through two small parallel incisions in the skin. Surgical success depends on the amount of apocrine gland that is removed.

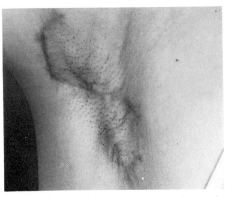

A good result after excision incorporating a z plasty.

Hydradenitis suppurativa

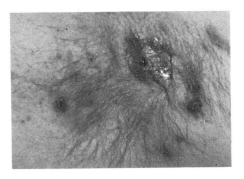

Hydradenitis suppurativa is an inflammatory disease of the apocrine sweat glands producing deep and recurring abscesses in the axilla. It is painful and causes a great deal of distress because of the discharging abscesses. Treatment initially is with appropriate broad spectrum antibiotics. Once the disease pattern has become established, however, most patients are grateful for surgical intervention. This consists of excising the whole area affected by the disease. Although large areas of skin may be excised from the axilla, skin grafts and local flaps may be required. The appreciable local discomfort and decreased abduction in the axilla caused by the scarring are far preferable to the symptoms of the disease. The groin and perineum may also be affected.

Xanthelasma

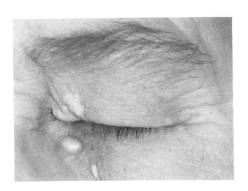

Xanthelasma presents most commonly in the form of soft, thin, elongated plaques, yellow and slightly raised in profile. They are often symmetrically distributed around the eyes and are common in the medial canthal area. In about half of all cases these lesions are associated with hyperlipoproteinaemia. In many cases, however, there is no apparent associated general disturbance of lipid metabolism and the xanthelasma is therefore just a simple, local, cosmetic problem. The xanthelasma may be excised surgically or eradicated with a topical sclerosant such as phenol. Patients should be screened for hyperlipoproteinaemia and referred to a physician should any abnormalities be found.

MALIGNANT SKIN CONDITIONS

Unlike most other examples of surgical pathology, malignant skin conditions can be diagnosed accurately from the history of the complaint combined with a thorough examination of the lesion under a good light with magnification. Skin cancer is the second most common tumour in men and women in the United Kingdom, accounting for just over 10% of all known malignancies or roughly 190 000 new cases a year.

The following symptoms may indicate malignancy: (1) a recent rapid appearance of or change in a long standing lesion; (2) a lesion that ulcerates or has periods of apparent healing fluctuating with either scabbing or ulceration; (3) itching caused by desquamation of cells; and (4) pain, which is less common but may indicate perineural infiltration.

Keratosis

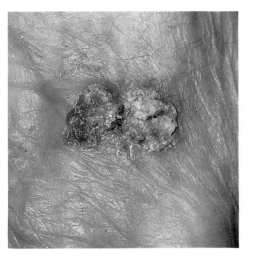

Excessive exposure to the sun leads to actinic damage. The skin protects itself by producing melanin and keratin. If the melanin response is poor, as it is in people with fair skin, or there are fewer melanocytes, as in older people, hyperkeratinisation and keratosis may develop. Clinically keratosis presents as a raised, scaly, erythematous lesion. Induration around the lesion may suggest malignant change. Metastases from subsequent carcinomas are rare. Arsenic keratoses present as punctate hyperkeratoses, often found on the palms and soles. They usually arise many years after systemic or topical exposure. The keratoses themselves seldom require treatment. They may, however, become malignant, and the patient should be examined regularly for this change and also for systemic malignancies.

In the treatment of multiple keratoses fluorouracil cream may helpful. The patient applies the cream night and morning under close medical supervision. The reaction begins on about the fifth day, producing an erythematous crusting, sometimes with superficial ulceration. When use of the cream is stopped vaseline should be applied to the treated area.

Bowen's disease

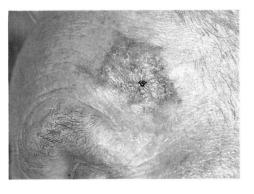

Bowen's disease presents as a chronic, nodular, intraepidermal plaque, which may ulcerate or become crusted. It may be associated with actinic damage or contact with arsenic. Histologically it is an intraepidermal squamous cell carcinoma that may occasionally become invasive. The diagnosis of such a lesion may be confirmed by excision biopsy. Treatment can be completed by surgical removal or, in selected cases, by cryotherapy or radiotherapy. In patients who have been excessively exposed to the sun avoidance of further actinic damage is important.

Malignant skin conditions

Keratoacanthoma

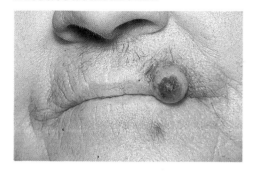

A keratoacanthoma is a dome shaped, umbilicated lesion with a central crater filled with keratin. It commonly develops on an exposed site in elderly people. It begins as a nodule, which grows steadily over several weeks and involutes spontaneously within a few months, leaving a depressed scar. True keratoacanthomas can therefore be left to heal spontaneously, but some are excised for cosmetic reasons. A proportion of apparent keratoacanthomas are, however, really squamous cell carcinomas and therefore need surgical excision. The treatment of these lesions requires experience and fine judgment.

Leukoplakia

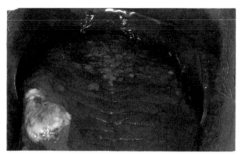

Leukoplakia is a condition of the mouth commonly occuring in middle aged and elderly patients. It especially affects smokers and those who have had chronic irritation of the mouth, often produced by ill fitting dentures. Clinically an area of the mucosa is covered with white raised multiple plaques. Those that are indurated and have fissures may progress to squamous cell carcinoma. The diagnosis should be confirmed histologically; treatment is then by either surgical excision or physical ablation, using the laser or cryoprobe, and correction of any predisposing factor. A similar pathological condition may affect the glans penis and vulva.

Hutchinson's melanotic freckle

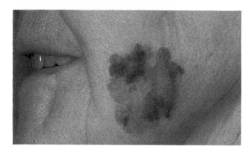

This lesion characteristically occurs on the face but may also be seen on the neck, back, or elsewhere on the body. The lesion is usually an irregular pigmented flat macule that grows slowly over 10 to 15 years. The lesion may proceed to a superficial malignant melanoma, which can present clinically as thickening of the lesion, a change in pigmentation, or itching. Prophylactic excision is the best treatment as it also permits histological examination.

Malignant conditions

Clinical types of basal cell carcinoma

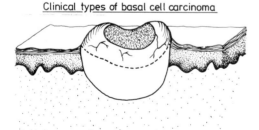

Nodular

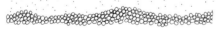

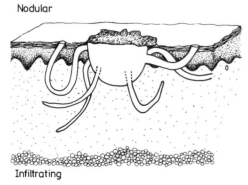

Infiltrating

Basal cell carcinoma

Basal cell carcinoma (or rodent ulcer) usually develops on hair bearing skin, mainly on the exposed areas of the head and neck. Roughly 30% of cases are multiple. A typical lesion is the nodular basal cell carcinoma, which has a pearly edge in which superficial blood vessels are visible. This well circumscribed tumour can be treated by surgical excision, radiotherapy, or other physical means of ablation such as laser or cryoprobe. Whatever method is used, the cure rate is extremely high at 95% or better.

Less common presentations of basal cell carcinoma may occur and include: the pigmented basal cell carcinoma, which can be confused with malignant melanoma; field fire lesion, a form of rodent ulcer that destroys a large area of skin in a short time and presents a major reconstructive problem after excision; and the more infiltrating type of tumour, the edge of which tends to be indistinct and the irradication of which may be incomplete or difficult because of diffuse dissemination through the local tissues. Treatment of this sort of tumour, particularly when situated around the eye, ear, or nose, may result in mutilating excisions. For the plastic surgeon, however, surgical reconstruction is easier when there has not been previous radiotherapy in these areas.

Most rodent ulcers do not metastasise, remaining a purely local problem. It is not possible to be dogmatic about whether they are best treated by surgery or radiotherapy. Before any particular form of treatment is decided on consideration should be given to the age and fitness of the patient, the type and site of basal cell carcinoma, and the local resources that are available to treat the patient.

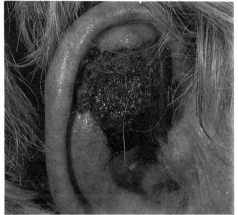

Squamous cell carcinoma.

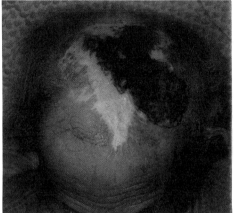

Marjolin ulcer in burn scar.

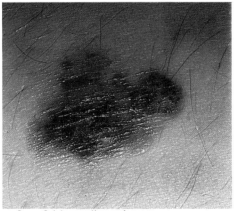

Superficial spreading melanoma.

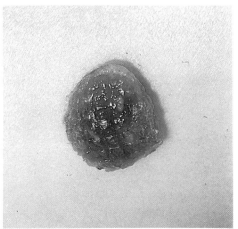

Nodular melanoma.

Squamous cell carcinoma

Squamous cell carcinomas are less common than rodent ulcers. Clinically they can present as: a hyperkeratosis with induration; an ulcer beneath a crusting surface; a persistent ulcer of the skin; an extension from a carcinoma of a deeper structure, such as a fungating maxillary sinus carcinoma; or a Marjolin ulcer (develops in an old, unstable scar).

Treatment again revolves around either surgery or radiotherapy. In general, excision of the squamous cell carcinoma should have a wider margin than that for less malignant basal cell carcinoma. Radiotherapy is of particular importance as an adjunct to surgery when there has been incomplete clearance, recurrence, or perineural spread of the tumour. These tumours do metastasise to the lymph nodes, but the incidence of such behaviour is low, being about 5% in actinic induced tumours but rising to about 15% in the Marjolin type ulcer. The treatment of the regional lymph nodes is usually by surgical excision, although in old and infirm patients radiotherapy may be preferred. The prognosis is related to the length of time the lesion has been present and its depth of invasion into the dermis; the deeper the invasion the more likely the tumour will be to metastasise.

Malignant melanoma

Malignant melanoma is the most serious of skin cancers and often affects young adults. Its incidence has doubled in the past 20 years in the United Kingdom, and roughly 2000 new cases now develop annually. Three quarters of all cases can be diagnosed clinically. Any pigmented lesion or mole that has recently appeared or changed must be considered suspicious. Particular attention should be given to any change in size or colour or to the development of itching or bleeding. The presence or absence of hair in the lesion is not important, but the loss of hair from a previously hairy mole may be relevant.

Presentation—Clinically there are four forms of presentation: a melanoma arising in a Hutchinson's melanotic freckle; a superficial spreading melanoma, which can develop on any part of the body and is the most common presentation; a nodular melanoma, which is the most malignant form; and the far rarer acral lentiginous melanoma occurring on plantar and palmar skin.

Prognosis—Sunlight is an important aetiological agent. The incidence of malignant melanoma in light skinned, fair haired people increases towards the equator. These people are particularly at risk if they have a lot of freckles and tend on exposure to the sun to burn rather than produce a tan. Several prognostic factors have been identified. Female patients survive longer than males. Lesions of the trunk, head, and neck have a worse prognosis than those affecting the arms and legs. Pathologically the depth of invasion may be related to prognosis. The older Clarke's classification, which related survival to depth of invasion into the layers of the dermis, has been superseded by a direct measurement of the thickness of the tumour. Breslow found that almost all patients with skin tumours thinner than 0·75 mm survived free from their disease for five or more years whereas lesions of greater thickness had a worse prognosis. Tumours thicker than 4·5 mm have only a 50% five year survival rate. Malignant melanoma disseminates via the dermal lymphatics to the regional lymph nodes. Once this has occurred the disease tends to run a relentlessly progressive course, and half such patients are dead within a year. Although spontaneous regression has been documented, it is rare.

Malignant skin conditions

Classification by depth of invasion.

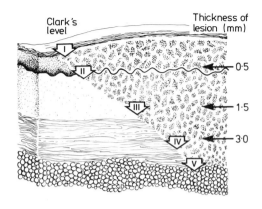

Sites of metastases (in order of presentation)

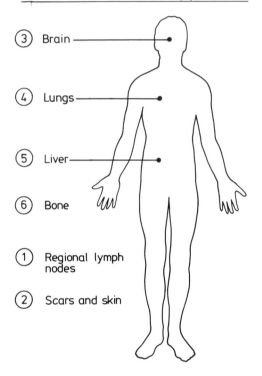

③ Brain

④ Lungs

⑤ Liver

⑥ Bone

① Regional lymph nodes

② Scars and skin

Treatment of malignant melanoma has recently undergone reappraisal. The classic treatment by wide excision and skin grafting for all melanomas was based on the evidence of a paper written over 50 years ago describing the treatment of a single case of recurrent melanoma in the groin rather than the treatment of a primary tumour. Any suspicious skin lesion should be excised with a clearance of at least 0·5 cm of normal skin and preferably by the widest possible skin margin consistent with primary skin closure. There is no evidence that an excision biopsy alters the prognosis and it allows an accurate histological diagnosis including measurement of the thickness of the tumour. Some surgeons now consider that for thin tumours (less than 0·75 mm) no further surgery is required and only the thicker tumours require the more classic wide excision, which includes a circumference of at least 5 cm of normal skin. Wide excisions may influence local recurrence, with an incidence of up to 10% for the thick lesions, but it probably does not influence the ultimate survival. Prophylactic dissection of lymph nodes is not generally undertaken in this country, but there may be an indication for it in thicker tumours on the arms and legs where the lesion is adjacent to the regional lymph nodes. Block dissections of the regional lymph nodes are otherwise undertaken only when these are clinically affected.

Advanced disseminated disease—In advanced disseminated disease other forms of treatment may help. Immunotherapy, and particularly the use of BCG vaccine, has not been of any overall, systemic benefit but intralesionally it may effect some control of dermal metastases. More recently, it has become evident that radiotherapy can provide good palliation, particularly in inoperable metastatic lymph nodes, symptomatic deposits in bone, or localised cerebral metastases. Chemotherapy can be used in two ways. Firstly, by regional perfusion for locally disseminated disease in an arm or leg and its regional lymph nodes. Its effect can be enhanced by hyperthermia. Such treatment can help to control local disease but has no effect on the overall survival and in some cases has been associated with a high incidence of complications. Secondly, systemic chemotherapy has been used. A single agent, in particular (DTIC (dimethyl triazine imidazole carboxemide) can induce remission in about 20% of cases, but this effect is usually short lived. More recently, other agents, particularly vindesine and cisplatin, have been tried either alone or in combination. As a generalisation, chemotherapy, while remaining the only hope for widespread disseminated disease, remains objectively unsubstantiated as a treatment especially when the serious side effects of the treatment and the low response rate are taken into consideration. It may be that chemotherapy should be used earlier in the disease in those patients who have a bad prognosis but no clinical evidence of dissemination.

Actinic damage and its treatment

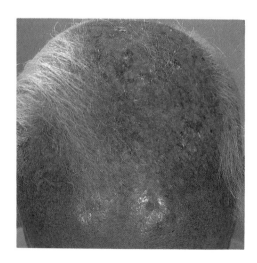

There is little doubt that repeated exposure to sunlight is a major factor in the development of many skin cancers. The skin's natural protection is to increase the thickness of the stratum corneum and produce pigment. Black skin is 10 times better than white skin at stopping ultraviolet light penetrating the full thickness of the epidermis. Ultraviolet B light (320-280 nm) is the wavelength of light that is responsible for producing tumours by a direct action on the basal layer cells of the epidermis. Ultraviolet A light (400-320 nm) is responsible for producing a tan by stimulating the melanocytes; this provides only limited protection to the basal layer from ultraviolet B.

The relative amount of ultraviolet B in the sun's rays is lessened by increases in the amount of atmospheric ozone. Thus less ultraviolet light traverses the atmosphere in the early and late parts of the day, when the rays pass obliquely through the atmosphere, compared with at midday, when the sun is overhead and the rays pass perpendicularly through the atmosphere. Clouds in the sky disrupt more of the ultraviolet A than the ultraviolet B and therefore give a false sense of security.

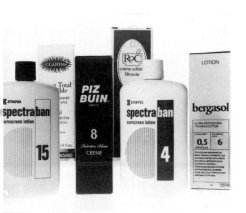

Protection from the sun's rays can be achieved by:

(1) *Clothing*—A hat provides cover for the face only down to the level of the nose and is usually worn by people who have already sustained actinic damage. The amount of protection from clothing depends on the weave of the fabric and will be relatively low for a woman wearing a light, cotton dress.

(2) *Glass and plastic*—Hard glass in particular acts as a poor filter. Perspex absorbs ultraviolet B strongly but does not provide an appreciable barrier to ultraviolet A.

(3) *Ultraviolet absorbent sun screens*—All commercially available sun screens contain substances that selectively absorb ultraviolet radiation. Their efficiency is expressed as the sun protection factor. The higher the factor number the better the protection. Such preparations as Spectraban 15, Coppertone Supershade 15, and ROC Total Sunblock Cream 10 are regarded as drugs and may therefore be prescribed in the normal way for certain skin conditions. Sun screen agents should be applied well before the start of perspiration. Unavoidable inaccuracy in application will lead to some areas being better protected than others. The liberal use of a poor sun screen is better than the conservative use of a powerful one spread thinly.

CHRONIC SWELLING OF THE LEG AND STASIS ULCER

Swelling of the leg is a condition often seen in general practice. Most commonly it develops secondarily to a local abnormality in the venous or lymphatic system, but systemic abnormalities such as cardiac or renal failure or myxoedema should not be overlooked.

By definition oedema is a pathological accumulation of fluid in the interstitial tissues. Physiologists divide the body water into intracellular and extracellular compartments, extracellular compartments consisting of the vascular circulation, lymphatic circulation, and interstitial "fluid." The interstitial fluid is a thin layer of gel, a colloidal system in which particles of solid are dispersed in a liquid. The interstitial compartment has a capacity to imbibe water but any such tendency is opposed by the osmotic pressure of the plasma, drawing water into the capillaries. The viability of cells is maintained by the continuously occurring transit of plasma fluid into the interstitial spaces (outward filtration) and back again (inward filtration). This transcapillary fluid exchange is in perfect balance under normal conditions. If this balance is disturbed the sol phase of the colloid increases its volume and oedema arises.

Extracellular fluid (15 l) = coordinated system of three compartments

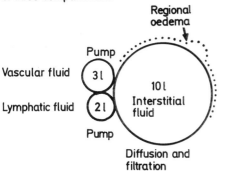

Oedema of venous origin

More than 90% of swollen legs seen in general practice result from incompetence of the venous system. This reversible orthostatic oedema (oedema arising after standing and disappearing when the venous perfusion pressure is lowered by raising the foot) is considered to be a dominating sign of impaired venous drainage of the leg. The terms varicose veins and epifascial chronic venous insufficiency are used when the pathology is limited to the superficial veins alone and the post thrombotic syndrome and deep chronic venous insufficiency when the oedema is induced by thrombosis of the deep veins.

Three clinical groups of patients presenting with varicose veins can be identified according to the severity of their signs and symptoms.

Clinical classification of varicose veins			
Type	Veins		
	Epifascial	Perforating	Deep
I Asymptomatic	Abnormal (+)	Normal	Normal
II Symptomatic	Abnormal (++)	Abnormal (+)	Normal
III With trophic change:			
Epifascial	Abnormal (+++)	Abnormal (+++)	Normal
Subfascial	Abnormal (+++)	Abnormal (+++)	Abnormal (+/+++)

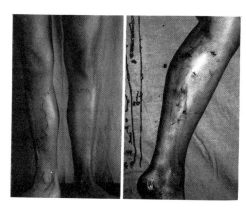

(1) *Asymptomatic varicose veins*—In most patients with varicose veins (even gross ones) the orthostatic oedema is so mild that it is of little clinical concern. These patients represent a well defined and easily treated group. The signs are of cosmetic relevance alone, and the therapeutic results after a simple stripping operation or injection of a sclerosant are excellent. A further common cosmetic complaint is the presence of spider veins, which tend to develop in the upper thigh and are very fine cutaneous venules. These are best treated by microinjections using a 26 G needle and taking care that only a small amount of weak sclerosant is used; otherwise unsightly pigmentation may occur.

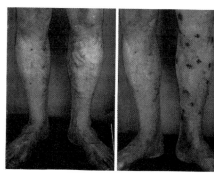

(2) *Symptomatic varicose veins*—The second group includes patients with complaints such as a feeling of heaviness, itching, tension, or cramps, or a combination of these, in the affected leg together with visible orthostatic oedema. Injection sclerotherapy usually gives poor long term results, and recurrence is common after the conventional stripping operation. The most common reason for this is the presence of several pathologically dilated muscle perforating veins or of an incompetent short saphenous vein that may not have been dealt with adequately at the first operation.

(3) *Varicose veins with trophic changes*—These patients display the highest morbidity. Their condition is characterised by the presence of trophic changes ranging from induration of the subcutaneous tissue to pigmentation, skin atrophy, and ulceration. Usual but not obligatory is impairment of both the deep and superficial venous drainage systems. Irrespective of the aetiology, the most important pathological factor is, in addition to epifascial varicosities, a vastly increased number of incompetent transfascial communicating veins resulting in severe dysfunction of the foot and calf muscle pumps. The swollen leg with extensive trophic changes responds poorly to compression treatment as well as to injection sclerotherapy and often recurs after conventional stripping operations. Satisfactory long term results can best be achieved from a dorsal subfascial approach, raising a long medial and lateral fasciocutaneous flap and ligating all dilated incompetent perforating veins.

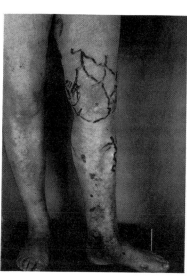

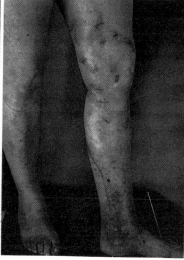

Oedema of lymphatic origin

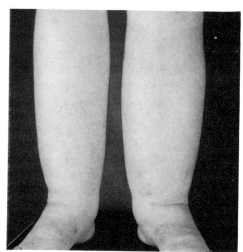

This form of swelling results from impaired transport of lymph, which arises either spontaneously (primary lymphoedema) or secondarily to damage of the lymphatic system, most often in Britain after surgical exenteration of the regional lymph nodes (secondary lymphoedema). Lymphoedema is typically unilateral but if it is bilateral it is always asymmetrical and has from the beginning little tendency to reversibility: when the patient gets up in the morning the leg is still swollen.

Chronic swelling of the leg and stasis ulcer

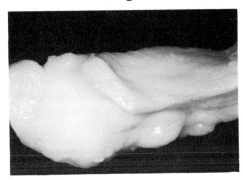

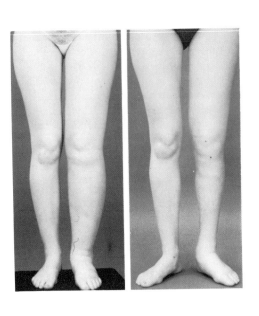

Lymphoedema, like venous oedema, is due to the overaccumulation of fluid in the interstitial spaces, but, whereas in venous oedema this is due to a pathological increase of intracapillary pressure, in lymphoedema it is related to an increased protein content in the interstitial fluid. In contrast to chronic venous insufficiency, the morphological changes induced by lymphatic impairment usually result in progressive increase in the girth of the affected extremity without clinically evident damage to the skin. The trophic changes, consisting mainly in severe fibrosis of the subcutaneous tissue and thickening of the fascia, have two important therapeutic consequences:

(1) The effect of externally applied pressure to the subcutis is considerably reduced (in severe fibrosis only 10% of the externally applied pressure may reach the subcutis).

(2) Compression treatment can effectively treat the overaccumulation of water but cannot reduce the enlarged girth due to fibrosis.

Nevertheless, the basic treatment for lymphoedema is compression treatment. It consists of the combined application of external intermittent compression by an electric pump and continuous compression by an elastic stocking of adequate compression grade. In advanced forms of lymphoedema with severe fibrosis of the skin and subcutaneous tissue the only effective treatment to reduce the girth is surgery. The operations performed in the past 80 years have aimed at either the improvement of lymph flow—drainage operations—or the reduction of the girth—excisional operations. In our hands all drainage operations have turned out to be unsatisfactory. The only operation consistently giving good long term results in both primary and secondary lymphoedema is the staged resection of the subcutaneous tissue along with thickened fascia and preservation of skin in the form of thin flaps. The operation improves the appearance of the leg, maintains the massage effect of the underlying muscles on the skin and makes the patient responsive to less vigorous compression treatment.

Lipoedema

> Characteristics of patients
>
> Stove pipe legs
> Jodhpur distribution of fat
> Small breasts
> No oedema of foot dorsum

Lipoedema, or lipidosis, occurs predominantly in young women and is characterised by bilateral moderate enlargment of the legs, without oedema, in the presence of normal veins and normal or minimally hypoplastic lymph ducts. Characteristically the patient has small breasts, a jodhpur distribution of fat in the thighs, large legs (stove pipe leg), and no oedema of the dorsum of the foot. The only available treatment that can be recommended is liposuction of the fat accumulation in the thighs.

Stasis ulcers

> Categories
>
> (1) Respond well to treatment
> 60%
>
> (2) Respond badly to treatment
> 40%

Most chronic ulcers of the leg are of venous origin. The immediate cause is a break down of the microcirculation with inadequate oxygenation of the affected area of skin. The typical site of a venous ulcer is above the medial malleolus, and, according to the "blow out" concept, they result from the incompetence of a supramalleolar ankle perforating vein. Many patients, however, with grossly dilated and incompetent ankle perforating veins have no trophic changes of the gaiter area whatsoever. In our experience a simultaneous dilatation and incompetence of all the main longitudinal veins along with most of the perforating veins is necessary for the development of an ulcer and its persistence.

Chronic swelling of the leg and stasis ulcer

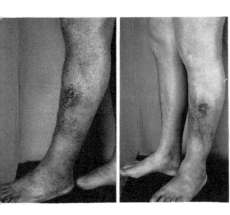

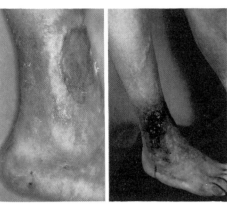

With regard to treatment chronic venous ulcers may be divided into two categories: those (60%) that respond well to treatment and those (40%) that do not. In those that respond well the ulcer develops above a cushion of dilated veins one of which is usually but not necessarily a perforating vein. Once these veins have been eliminated by compression, injection, or surgery the ulcer heals spontaneously or more rapidly with a partial thickness skin graft. This skin graft should remain supported by adequate elasticated compression from the toes to the knee at all times when the leg is dependent postoperatively.

In ulcers that do not respond well the dependence on dilated veins is not evident and the main pathophysiological factor is severe dysfunction of the calf muscle pump. This in turn results from several factors occurring in various combinations. They are: an increased number of incompetent communicating veins; varicosities of both long and short saphenous veins; a restricted range of movement at the ankle and metatarsal joints; and a "chronic compartment syndrome" due to the induration of epifascial tissues. The treatment of choice is the improvement of the muscle pump effect by a subfascial operation ligating incompetent perforating veins combined with skin grafting of the ulcer.

Less often the cause of non-healing is mycotic infection, a lowered resistance to infection by the patient, or arterial insufficiency. More rarely ulcers may be of tuberculous or syphilitic origin or a complication of systemic diseases such as ulcerative colitis. It should also be borne in mind that malignancy can occur in long standing ulcers and that a biopsy should therefore be performed whenever there is doubt about the diagnosis.

COSMETIC SURGERY: THE AGING FACE

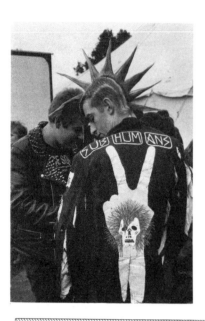

Four types of abnormality	
	Example
1 Congenital	Protruding ears
2 Abnormal development	Disproportional breast growth
3 Post-traumatic	Scars of the face
4 Normal aging	Bags round the eyes

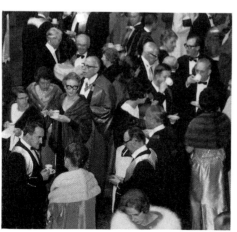

Conforming display.

Display is an important animal instinct, which may manifest itself in primitive societies by body adornment with various dyes or elaborate scars and even more drastic anatomical changes such as increasing the size of the lips or the lobes of the ears. Our own society's equivalents include tattooing the wearing of makeup and jewellery, and the changing of hair styles. This may be reinforced for many of us by the wish to conform with our peers or with the demands of society. It seems that in all of us there are behavioural patterns or instincts to alter or promote our appearance.

Recently a concept of aestheticality has been introduced: just as some people are musical, so others have a highly developed sense of body image and thus are more motivated to have any abnormality in their appearance corrected. Abnormalities may be produced in one of four ways (table). Whichever way an abnormality arises, many people can compensate satisfactorily. Others, however, undergo immense psychological distress as a result of their perceived appearance, and this may be exacerbated by teasing at school or at work or by the pressures of contemporary advertising which equates youth and beauty with money, success, and happiness.

The reason why some people request cosmetic surgery when others with an apparently identical problem do not is, however, difficult to understand for cosmetic surgery is often sought by attractive people with slight imperfections as well as by people with gross abnormalities. Detailed psychological assessments of patients requesting cosmetic surgery have shown many to be at the hysterical end of the spectrum of normal personalities. This does not mean that patients who fall into this group should not be treated by cosmetic surgery for often this may work out more satisfactory and cheaper than treating them with drugs or psychotherapy over a long period. Indeed, cosmetic surgeons have been called psychiatrists who treat patients with a scalpel rather than with drugs.

For many cosmetic surgery may be an acceptable treatment for overcoming a personal crisis, and without doubt such patients if properly referred by a sympathetic general practitioner may be helped by cosmetic surgery. Unfortunately, some patients think they cannot get a sympathetic hearing from their general practitioner and therefore refer themselves directly to a plastic surgeon or to a financially motivated clinic that advertises. Cosmetic surgery is no longer only for the rich and famous or the obsessive and neurotic. It is a service demanded by the public and is justifiable on social, psychological, and maybe even economic grounds and should therefore be available through the National Health Service as well as privately.

There is one type of patient to avoid operating on. This is the dysmorphophobic, who is psychotic and becomes besotted with one part of his or her body and can never be satisfied no matter how excellent the surgery undertaken. These patients can become extremely disturbed.

Cosmetic surgery of the aging face

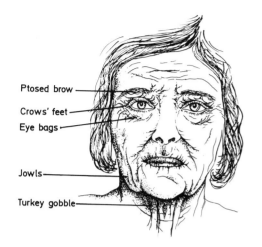

Ptosed brow

Crows' feet

Eye bags

Jowls

Turkey gobble

All structures in the body, including the skin and underlying facial muscles, age. The epidermis becomes flatter with a decreased turnover of cells. The major changes are in the dermis, which becomes thinner because of the loss of collagen and fluid and where, in addition, a decrease in the cross linkage of the collagen fibres is accompanied by a loss of elastin fibres. Thus the skin develops a fixed laxity rather than the reversible extensibility of youth. Muscle weakness results in wrinkles and deep creases at the points of greatest mobility—that is, around the eyes and mouth. This, together with the normal centripetal redistribution of fat, results in prominent accumulations around the eyelids, because of weakness of the obicularis muscle, and around the angle of the jaw, forming jowls, because of the weakness in the platysma.

Blepharoplasty

The eyes are important in communication and are said to reflect a person's inner being. The essential features of the aging process that affect them are:

(1) Ptosis of the eyebrows due to a weak frontalis muscle. Women disguise this by plucking hair from the lower part of the eyebrow and reinforcing the upper part with a pencil.

(2) Excess skin, particularly in the upper eyelid. When the brow is raised this may be less apparent. To a lesser extent excess skin may also develop in the lower eyelid.

(3) Herniation of fat, through the weak obicularis muscle, producing bags, particularly in the medial canthus of the upper lid and in the whole of the lower lid. There may be a familial predisposition to forming baggy eyelids, and this is usually more apparent early in the day. In younger people bagginess may be produced in the lower eyelids by hypertrophy of the obicularis muscle, and in these cases there may not be an excess accumulation of fat.

(4) The development of creases ("crows' feet") radiating out from the lateral canthus.

Before undertaking surgery the physical problem must be diagnosed exactly. Important medical causes of oedema of the eyelids should be eliminated, visual acuity assessed, and the presence of normal tear secretion and drainage checked. In older patients laxity in the lower lid margin with early ectropion should be looked for with care. Both lifting of the brow and reduction of the eyelids may be done under local anaesthesia with sedation on a day case principle or under general anaesthesia.

Brow lift is done through a coronal incision set well back in the hair and undermining down to the supraorbital rim. The forehead is then pulled upwards, taking care to preserve the cutaneous nerves and excising the procerus muscle overlying the glabella area of the nose. The scalp is sutured after excision of the appropriate amount. In general, the procedure is free from complications (apart from the development in some cases of an anaesthetic area in the central forehead). It can appreciably improve the appearance of the eyes.

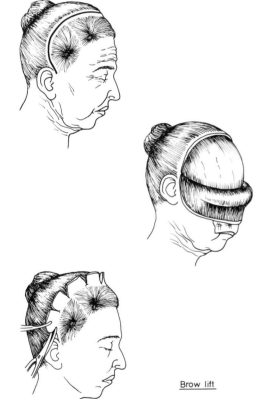

Brow lift

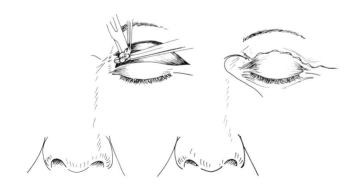

Upper eyelid reduction is performed by excising an ellipse of skin from the upper lid together with excess fat from the medial canthal region—a procedure free from complications provided care is taken.

41

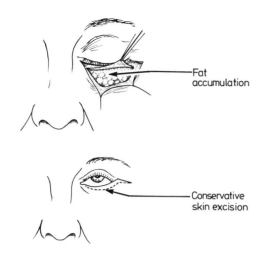

Fat accumulation

Conservative skin excision

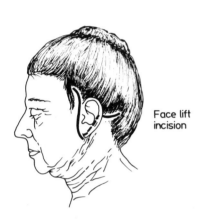

Face lift incision

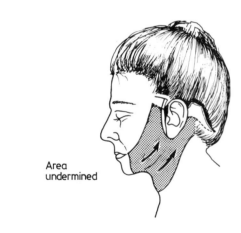

Area undermined

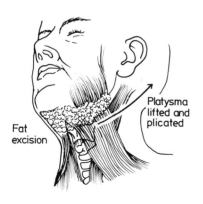

Fat excision

Platysma lifted and plicated

Lower eyelid reduction is done through an incision along the tarsal plate just below the eyelashes and extending out laterally into the crows' feet. Excess fat causing the bags is removed as, at the same time, is any excess skin. This particular procedure requires extreme skill as it is a delicate balance between excising enough skin to produce the desired cosmetic improvement and not producing an ectropion. Many patients who have had the right amount of skin excised initially have a minimal ectropion, often due to postoperative oedema, which settles within a week. Occasionally too much fat may be excised producing a rather cachectic look, and this obviously requires judgment. The ultimate complication of blindness occurs in one in 500 000 cases. It is caused by a retrobulbar haematoma, which if diagnosed early can be relieved. The fine creases are not altered, but it is a good procedure for dealing with bags in the lower lids.

Rhytidectomy

With weakening of the platysma muscle the support to the neck and chin region is lost. Fat becomes redistributed in the face causing jowls to develop in the cervicomandibular area and, in the more obese, a submental collection of fat. The platysma muscle can also form into folds under the chin, producing a so called turkey gobble.

In the standard face lift operation a preauricular incision extending around the back of the ear is continued perpendicularly into the posterior scalp at a height well covered by hair. The skin is then mobilised as a large flap via this incision forwards almost to the nasolabial fold and downwards towards the midline of the neck in a plane superficial to the platysma muscle to avoid damaging the facial nerve. In some patients a submental incision is required to facilitate excision of fat in this area. Any excess fat lying superficial to the platysma muscle can be excised with obvious benefit to the jowls. At the same time the platysma muscle is repositioned by redraping its posterior border and hitching it up high onto the sternomastoid muscles just under the ear. This recreates a sharper angle at the junction of the neck and submental area. Not all patients, however, require this surgery to the platysma.

In general, the standard face lift does little for the mid-face and nothing for the creases in the upper lip. Its major indication is for the neck region, where gratifying results can be achieved. Smaller procedures such as "minilifts" may produce an initial improvement, but experience has shown that these are not sustained. As described it is not a minor procedure, and I think it as best done under general anaesthesia with a stay of two to three days in hospital.

As for any surgery, there are complications. Three per cent of patients have large haematomas requiring drainage, and roughly 15% have small haematomas, which resolve spontaneously. Between one and five per cent of patients sustain sensory nerve injury, most commonly to the greater auricular nerve supplying the lower part of the ear. More importantly, in up to 2% of cases the facial nerve may be damaged. This is usually a neuropraxia, and the most common branches injured are the cervicomandibular branch and the branch to the frontalis. Scars in front of the ear heal well. The scar extending horizontally behind the ear sustains the main brunt of tension in a face lift and often has areas of minor necrosis and quite obvious hatch marks, which are produced by the skin sutures. Fortunately this scar should be covered by normal hair growth provided it is positioned high enough in the scalp.

This operation has now become far more common for men. In general, the results are less good than in women, and a higher motivation is required. The scars can be covered in front of the ears with lengthening side boards, but the growth of the beard behind the ears can be a problem.

I am often asked, "How long does the benefit from these procedures last?" Within the limitations of personal variation a face lift and eyelid reduction set the aging process back between seven and 10 years. Unfortunately, we all go on aging, and surgery will not alter the rate at which this occurs; it merely sets the clock back.

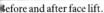

Before and after face lift.

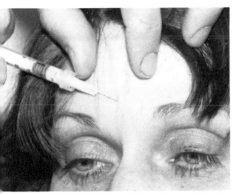

Collagen injection of crease.

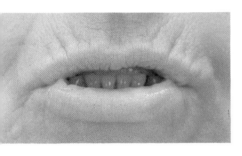

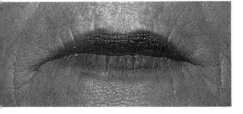

Skin creases

The more major deep creases, in particular the nasolabial fold and the crows' feet lateral to the eyes are not well managed by the operations described above. The recently introduced, injectible collagen goes some way to overcoming this problem. The bovine dermal collagen is treated by lyophilisation and manufactured in a saline suspension. After a test dose in the forearm to rule out the 2% of patients who are allergic to bovine protein the skin crease can be raised by a series of injections along it. Over correction is required as initially the saline is absorbed and over six months to a year there is a further relapse depending on the amount of collagen that is removed. Nevertheless, the procedure has a place in the cosmetic armamentarium.

The fine creases that occur particularly around the mouth and eyes are best treated by chemical peel or dermabrasion. In chemical peel a phenol solution is used to produce a chemical burn that causes a loss of the superficial epithelium without producing a full thickness burn. Experience is required in its application to avoid complications. It should be done as an inpatient procedure as initially the pain is severe. In most cases there is a satisfactory smoothing of the fine creases.

The major disadvantage is a change in the pigmentation. Initially there is hyperpigmentation caused by erythema, which matures to produce a hypopigmented scar. There is a danger that when the patient sits in the sun the pale area around the eyes and mouth will produce a panda look. This procedure is also best avoided in dark skinned people because of variable and unpredictable pigment changes.

Phenol can be absorbed through the skin, and extreme caution should be exercised with a total face peel as toxic concentrations of phenol can occur in the blood.

COSMETIC AND RECONSTRUCTIVE SURGERY OF THE BREAST

The most common breast deformities
for which surgery is sought

- Breast hypertrophy
- Breast hypoplasia
- Breast asymmetry
- Breast ptosis
- Postmastectomy deformity

Breasts come in different shapes, sizes, and degrees of symmetry and continue to change in the wake of pregnancy, fluctuations in body weight, aging, and breast disease. Women react in different ways to natural or pathological variations in breast form, and, though some may accept the deformity and scarring that follow radical mastectomy and radiotherapy for carcinoma of the breast, others will be unable to tolerate minor loss of breast shape and bulk after pregnancy and seek restoration. Given that restorative and reconstructive surgery of the breast is objectively not essential it can sometimes be difficult for a medical practitioner to sympathise with the motivation of a woman requesting surgery. Experience and sound psychological evaluation have, however, shown that plastic and reconstructive surgery of the breast in carefully selected and primed patients is an important and gratifying service.

Augmentation of the breast

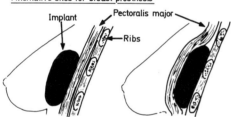

Alternative sites for breast prosthesis

Implant — Pectoralis major — Ribs

Augmentation of the breast in the treatment of breast hypoplasia is the commonest form of breast surgery. It is a simple and safe surgical procedure in which an appropriately sized silicone gel prosthesis is implanted to a submusculofascial pocket dissected between the chest wall and the pectoral muscles or to a pocket between the muscles and the breast tissue by a small incision made behind the anterior fold of the axilla, within the areola, or, most commonly, just above the submammary crease. The pocket is usually drained during the two days in hospital.

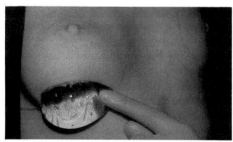

Insertion of silicone prosthesis via submammary incision.

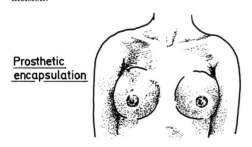

Prosthetic encapsulation

At body temperature the silicone has the consistency and mobility of normal breast tissue but, unfortunately, it has a natural tendency for encapsulation by a mesothelial lined membrane that, if sufficiently thick and fibrotic, transforms the breast into a hard, ugly, and tender sphere. This phenomenon of spherical fibrous contracture develops in about 10 to 20% of all women after augmentation of the breast. The thick capsule can be dispersed by manual compression under sedation or light anaesthesia ("breast popping") but may recur, in which case readmission to hospital becomes necessary to excise the capsule, redissect a larger pocket, and replant the prosthesis. There is no reliable means of predicting or preventing spherical fibrous encapsulation, but routine daily massage of the prosthesis to maintain the capacity of the dissected pocket does seem to reduce the incidence and should be continued for at least three months.

Cosmetic and reconstructive surgery of the breast

Reduction of the breast

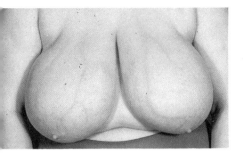

Very large breasts are not only a source of embarrassment but a cause of submammary intertrigo, postural compensation leading at a later age to cervical arthropathy and deep grooving of the shoulders as a consequence of the great weight suspended from the straps of a brassière. The technique of surgical reduction whereby a large sphere is converted to a smaller one is not easy to explain but basically requires the dismantling of the breast and excision of excess breast tissue and skin (routinely sent for histological examination) before resiting the nipple and areola complex and reassembling the remaining breast into a smaller and more manageable form.

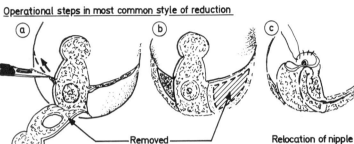

Operational steps in most common style of reduction

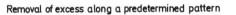

Removed

Relocation of nipple aureolar complex

Removal of excess along a predetermined pattern

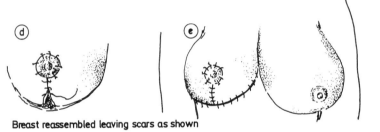

Breast reassembled leaving scars as shown

The price a woman has to pay is periareolar scarring together with an anchor shaped scar on the lower half of the breast and a nipple and areola that, as a result of being resited, may have altered erotic sensation as well as the guaranteed inability to act as a milk conduit having been detached from the underlying lactiferous ducts. (In particularly large breasts the nipple and areola are replaced as a free graft so that loss of breast feeding and sensation are inevitable.) The stay in hospital is around four days with interruption of normal daily routine for up to four weeks.

The early complications are dehiscence at the junction of the vertical and longitudinal component of the scar and infrequently partial loss of areola skin. Both these complications can be managed conservatively with the encouragement of secondary epithelialisation. A later and more persistent complication is called low grade fat necrosis: patchy and poorly diffused areas of the breast become lumpy and tender but gradually soften after a few months.

Mastopexy

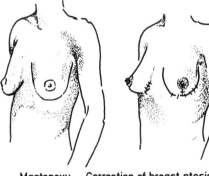

Mastopexy   Correction of breast ptosis without reduction of breast volume

The appearance post partum of ptotic, striae spattered breasts of reasonable volume may be improved by reducing the skin envelope, along the same lines as for a reduction of the breast, to leave an identical pattern of scarring except for a shorter length to the horizontal scar. As the breast tissue itself is not reduced the nipple and areola can be resited without being detached from the underlying ducts and glands, thus allowing a woman to breast feed at a later date. Having, however, acquired the original ptosis as a result of post lactational involution she is unlikely to go through another pregnancy. There is no effective surgical treatment for striae except including them within the excised areas of redundant breast skin during mastopexy. A woman has to come to terms with residual striae on the upper pole of the breast.

Developmental asymmetry of the breast

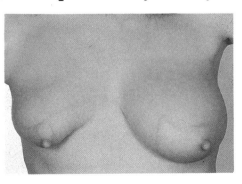

Minor degrees of asymmetry of the breast are common and virtually undetectable, but more obvious asymmetry, varying from Poland's syndrome to unequal breast size requiring some form of external padding, is not acceptable and deserves treatment. Poland's syndrome (the complete form is unilateral absence of breast and nipple and areola complex associated with a hypoplastic pectoralis major and ipsilateral anomalies of the hand) is managed along the lines of reconstruction of the breast after mastectomy, but other forms of asymmetry are treated by surgical augmentation or reduction of the relevant breast. In the knowledge of potential problems of spherical fibrous contracture after augmentation of the breast a surgeon is likely to try to sway a woman towards reduction of the larger breast to match the smaller one.

Cosmetic and reconstructive surgery of the breast
Reconstruction of the breast after mastectomy

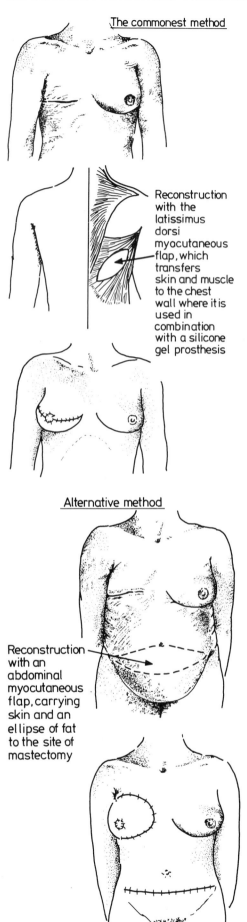

The commonest method

Reconstruction with the latissimus dorsi myocutaneous flap, which transfers skin and muscle to the chest wall where it is used in combination with a silicone gel prosthesis

Alternative method

Reconstruction with an abdominal myocutaneous flap, carrying skin and an ellipse of fat to the site of mastectomy

About 10% of women who undergo mastectomy afterwards have persistent serious anxiety, depression, or sexual problems that justify rehabilitation by reconstruction of a breast mound, and certain other women who are not so psychologically mutilated equally deserve reconstruction should they want it. Reconstruction is not, however, generally accepted to be advisable if the original tumour was staged at more than $T_2N_0M_0$, although some surgeons do not believe a more extensive breast carcinoma to be a contraindication.

Reconstruction is seldom planned before three months after the original mastectomy and is usually delayed for a year in the event of adjuvant radiotherapy. A few general surgeons, however, favour reconstruction at the same operation on the grounds that if the primary clearance of the tumour and affected glands is sufficiently radical the immediate introduction of flaps and prosthesis necessary for reconstruction can be done with sound justification.

Surgical reconstruction is essentially surgical arithmetic whereby structures lost during mastectomy are replaced in kind. Thus, after a simple mastectomy, when a sufficient volume of healthy skin and pectoral musculature remain, an internal silicone prosthesis can be inserted as for a cosmetic augmentation of the breast. After a radical mastectomy with associated radiotherapy, however, both bulk and healthy skin need to be replaced in the form of either a latissimus dorsi myocutaneous flap overlying a silicone prosthesis or a transposed abdominal flap that carries sufficient bulk of fat to obviate an internal prosthesis. (This property of the abdominal flap is particularly appealing as there is a built in bonus of a simultaneous abdominoplasty, but unfortunately the chances of flap necrosis are higher than with the use of a latissimus dorsi flap.)

Whatever technique is used, a breast cannot be replaced; the surgeon's goal is to construct a convincing mound that matches as nearly as possible the volume, position, and shape of the opposite breast and that permits the display of a balanced cleavage and equal filling of the cups of a brassière. Should the opposite breast be large or ptotic a compromise has to be reached in which the volume and shape of the normal breast is adjusted by reduction or mastopexy to meet the shape and size of the reconstructed breast. The possibilities, limitations, and "trade offs" in added scars in the course of reconstruction of the breast must therefore be clearly explained to a prospective patient, with the help of illustrations as required. If she has doubts about committing herself she should be advised against the operation as she is likely to be disappointed with the final result. Follow up shows, however, that informed and wholly committed patients are delighted with the planned outcome.

Surprisingly few women in Britain request reconstruction of the nipple and areola, which, if demanded, can be done either with the help of a graft from the opposite nipple and areola, if there is enough to spare, or as a tailored split skin graft harvested from the inner aspect of the thigh and draped over raised dermal flaps to give the projection of a simulated nipple. Alternatively, an adhesive nipple and areola prosthesis can be used to give the necessary "button" beneath the blouse or brassière.

COSMETIC SURGERY: OTHER PROCEDURES

Rhinoplasty

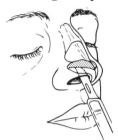

Alar cartilage reduction

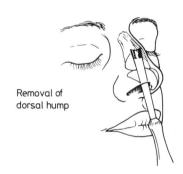

Removal of dorsal hump

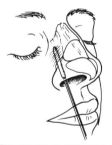

Fracturing of nasal bones

Rhinoplasty is the most popular of all cosmetic surgical procedures. The nose may be considered to require an overall reduction in size, or surgery may be sought to correct the shape of a normal sized nose—for example, if there is a large dorsal hump or the nose may have been damaged and either be crooked or have a depressed dorsal profile, possibly also with nasal airway obstruction. The surgeon must understand exactly what the patient is requesting before undertaking surgery, and preoperative photography may well help in this instance. The other important point to explain to the patient is that, although the surgeon's skill is important in the final outcome, so also is the way in which the patient's tissues heal. This is particularly important in the way a nose tip finally takes up its shape.

Standard rhinoplasty in this country is done under general anaesthesia. A bloodless surgical field is provided by either hypotensive anaesthesia or the injection of a weak adrenaline solution into the tissues of the nose. All incisions are made endonasally (inside the nose) except in very large noses that are being made considerably smaller, in which case the lateral alar bases are excised, leaving very fine scars at the junction of the nose with the nasolabial fold.

The basic procedures are:
(1) The dome of the alar cartilages is excised to make the tip of the nose smaller.
(2) A deviated septum is either resected or repositioned.
(3) The caudal end of the septum may be shortened.
(4) Surgery is then directed to the dorsum of the nose, which is partly cartilage, partly bone. It is usually reduced in height, but in some cases augmentation is required. A bone graft can be taken from the iliac crest or rib, cartilage from the rib or ear. Alternatively, silastic can be inserted into a pocket lying above the nasal septum to improve the dorsal profile.
(5) The nose is usually then made thinner by fracturing the nasal bones as they arise from the maxilla, and their position is held with a plaster of Paris splint.

The lining of the nose is carefully repaired and postoperative haemorrhage controlled with nasal packs, which are removed within the first 24 hours. The operation is not painful, but patients feel uncomfortable until the nasal packs are removed. The necessary orbital ecchymosis may be quite severe in the first 48 hours but completely resolves within two weeks, at which time the plaster of Paris is removed. The patient is usually in hospital for two to three days.

Despite careful surgery up to 20% of rhinoplasties may require a small secondary procedure, which can usually be done under local anaesthesia. A well performed rhinoplasty producing the desired result for the patient is one of the most satisfying procedures for a plastic surgeon to perform as it may produce changes in a patient's appearance and psyche for which he or she is extremely grateful.

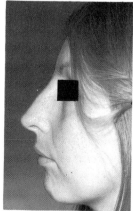

Before and after rhinoplasty.

Cosmetic surgery: other procedures
Reduction of the abdomen

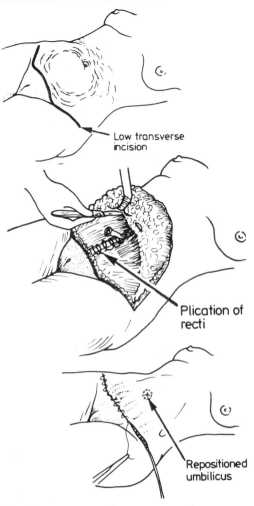

Low transverse incision

Plication of recti

Repositioned umbilicus

It is not known why some women who have multiple pregnancies can retain almost the same contour to their abdomen as they had in their younger days when others after a single pregnancy develop excess folds of skin that becomes thin and deeply marked with striae. At the same time excess adipose tissue may accumulate and the recti muscles become divarificated. Once such patients have undertaken to lose weight the situation can be greatly improved by excising the excess abdominal skin.

In the standard operation, performed under general anaesthesia, a low transverse incision is made in the area covered by the bikini bottom. Skin of the abdomen is mobilised virtually up to the costal margin and the umbilicus is circumcised, allowing it to be repositioned. The hole through which the umbilicus has been removed can in most cases be drawn down to the lower wound edge just above the pubic bones. Occasionally there is not enough excess skin, and a midline vertical scar is therefore necessarily produced. At the same time any divarification of the recti muscles can be corrected by plicating the rectus sheaths with a non-absorbable suture. The excess skin is then excised, leaving a low transverse incision and a further circular incision around the umbilicus.

In correctly selected patients this operation produces good results and gratified patients. Major short term complications are haematoma in roughly 2% of cases and minor skin breakdown in the incision line in the suprapubic area. Longer term complications include numbness in the midline and a rim of oedema above the transverse incision. Both of these symptoms usually settle without further treatment.

Body contouring operations

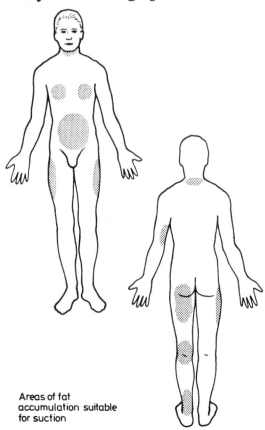

Areas of fat accumulation suitable for suction

Obese patients are best served by initial weight reduction followed by surgical excision of the excess skin. Skin and fat are sometimes in excess in the upper arms and the thighs. After weight reduction excess skin may drape off the upper arms and in some patients may present a distressing deformity when the patient abducts the arm to show two empty bags of skin. This excess skin can be excised, but the resulting scars are extremely unattractive and usually require the patient to keep this area permanently covered. The procedure, however, allows closer fitting clothes to be worn.

A similar condition can happen in the buttock and upper thigh region. Occasionally a procedure to lift the buttocks or upper thighs, or both, is indicated. By making an incision in the gluteal fold and extending it into the inguinal region and by undermining the upper thigh excess skin and fat can be excised. The scars are usually easily hidden, but again careful selection of patients is required.

Certain surgeons think that there are two types of subcutaneous fat. Firstly, there is the type that disappears with dieting, leaving the excess of skin as previously described. Secondly, there is a type that occurs mostly below the waist and is not influenced by dieting. The patient will therefore be left with an accumulation of fat in certain areas that no amount of dieting can remove. Such areas are over the greater trochanter, producing a sort of jodhpur effect; this may be removed by surgery alone and is best performed by a new procedure of fat suction. This procedure is indicated for localised accumulations of fat, particularly in younger patients. It is usually done under general anaesthesia. The area of fat accumulation is marked out carefully before the operation, which may be done as a dry procedure. Some practitioners inject a weak hypotonic saline solution to try to rupture the fat cell membranes, but this is not universal. A long metal cannula is

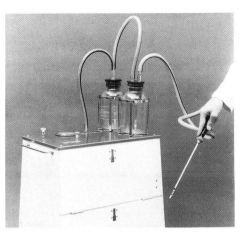

introduced through a small incision at a distance from the fat accumulation, and a strong negative pressure is provided by a suitable machine. Postoperatively, careful strapping of the treated area is required to provide topical pressure, and the patient can usually be discharged from hospital the next day.

Complications include repeated seroma production, uneven removal of fat, and a bevel at the edge of the treated area. This technique can be applied to other areas of fat accumulation in the lower abdomen, submentally in the neck, and to localised lipomas over the rest of the body.

Reassignment of gender

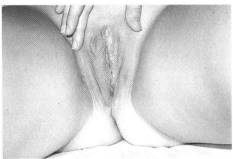

Male to female conversion.

There are an estimated 10 000 transsexuals in the United Kingdom, of whom about 1000 have received surgery of one form or another. Team management is required for this and is usually based around the psychiatrist to whom the patients are referred in the first instance. Initially, the patient has to live in the role of the new gender for at least two years, totally for the final year. This period may be reinforced with hormone treatment. At the same time, patients, particularly men becoming women, are instructed in the attitudes and mannerisms of the new sex so that they can fill the role more successfully.

It remains unproved whether psychotherapy, psychotrophic drugs, or surgery is the best long term treatment for this distressing group of patients. Any surgery that may be advocated by the psychiatrist is undertaken by a urologist or plastic surgeon. Most surgery is undertaken on the male to female gender reassignment, the most radical procedure being amputation of the genitals but using the penile and scrotal skin to line a newly created vagina. Other surgical procedures may include breast augmentation and facial surgery and of course electrolysis to try to irradicate hair from the beard.

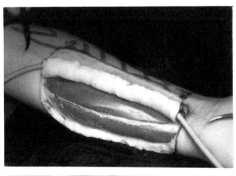

Female to male reassignment, apart from hysterectomy, bilateral mastectomy, and oophorectomy, is far more difficult. Until recently the only way to create any sort of penis was to use a tube pedicle or a local myocutaneous flap, requiring a multiple stage procedure with quite extensive local scarring to produce an organ which was in many instances unsatisfactory, usually because it was too large. More recently, radial forearm flaps have been adapted to allow a one or two stage construction of a phallus with a urethra. This is intended to provide the patient with an organ that allows him to stand with his colleagues and pass water in a public urinal and in no way is meant for sexual intercourse, in which case it would require reinforcement with a silastic rod.

This sort of surgery meets with a fair amount of scepticism from colleagues in general medicine and tends to be viewed completely unsympathetically. In carefully selected cases, however, who have been managed with the team approach, a well adjusted patient may be produced who can be reintegrated into society.

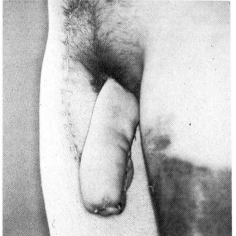

Phallus construction using radial forearm flap.

HEAD AND NECK CANCER

Causal factors
Leucoplakia
Age and sex
Cigarette and alcohol consumption
Chronic trauma
Betel nut and lime
Chronic sepsis
Actinic damage
Irradiation

Malignant tumours of the head and neck account for 2% of all cancers (excluding skin tumours). Treatment should aim at eradicating the cancer while, as far as possible, preserving physiological function and an acceptable appearance. This is not always possible; some tumours can be cured only at the cost of considerable morbidity.

Patients with head and neck cancer often delay seeking medical advice, sometimes through fear, sometimes through fecklessness. As prognosis is directly related to the stage of the disease at initial diagnosis delay should be minimised. In general terms, five year survival is 70% with localised disease but only 30% when disease has spread to the lymph nodes. Any lesion in the mouth that persists for three weeks without a tissue diagnosis should be biopsied. Hoarseness lasting longer than three weeks should be referred for specialist opinion.

Most head and neck tumours can be seen on careful clinical examination with a head light and mirror. There is a prognostic gradient that correlates with the ease with which a tumour can be visualised. Carcinomas of the lip, for example, have a better prognosis than carcinomas of the tongue. Tongue tumours, in turn, have a better prognosis than tumours of the hypopharynx. An exception to this is carcinoma of the larynx, which has a good prognosis, presumably because even a small tumour will produce noticeable hoarseness.

Important factors in treatment

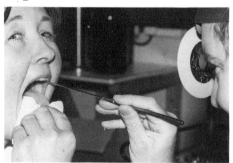

Examination using head light and mirror.

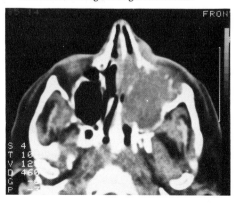

The patient

Important factors in the patient include his or her general health, previous treatment, social habits, and personality. Coincident medical conditions, such as chronic bronchitis, may preclude aggressive surgery, whereas alcoholics are often unreliable about attending for protracted courses of radiation treatment. All patients should be advised to stop smoking and to cut down, if not to eliminate, their consumption of alcohol.

The tumour

Treatment should not be started without histological proof of malignancy. The clinical stage and degree of histological differentiation of the tumour critically affect treatment and prognosis. The patient should be fully assessed (history, physical examination, examination under anaesthesia) so that the tumour can be assigned to the appropriate TNM category.

Patients with asymptomatic primary tumours and metastatic disease affecting critical organs should not be treated actively. If, however, metastatic disease is not immediately life threatening it may be necessary to treat the primary tumour actively to forestall the development of local symptoms. Patients with large primary tumours usually have distressing symptoms. Active treatment of the primary tumour is required, even though prognosis is poor, to restore some level of comfort to the patient.

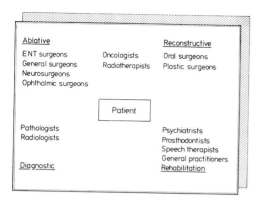

Head and neck cancers with variable pathology and sites of presentation do not generally fit into the domain of any one particular specialist. Formerly, if they were referred to the radiotherapist they were treated with radiotherapy; if referred to a surgeon they were treated surgically. Nowadays, the team approach allows for a better assessment of the patient and better rationalisation of treatment options. The team approach also allows for flexibility because if one modality is seen to be failing treatment can easily be changed. A team should ideally include all the following: a diagnostic or ablative surgeon (usually an ear, nose, and throat or general surgeon), a reconstructive surgeon, a radiotherapist/oncologist, and an oral surgeon. The team approach allows for a more critical analysis of results and avoids one specialty obtaining a biased view of another specialty's treatment by treating only that specialty's failures.

Treatment

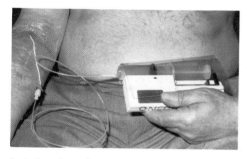

Ambulant chemotherapy.

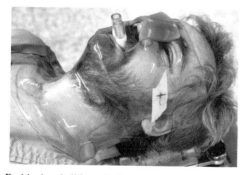

Positioning shell for radiotherapy.

Radiotherapy

Advantages

Good appearance and function

Treats large areas

Before operation: sterilises well oxygenated tumour cells at periphery of tumour

Disadvantages

Prolonged

Acute toxicity

Unpleasant

Long term taste change and dry mouth

Psychologically tumour not removed

Chemotherapy

Response rates of 50-80% can be obtained with chemotherapy for head and neck cancer, and these responses may translate into improved local control. Chemotherapy seems to have little effect in preventing growth or recurrence of systemic metastases and thus little influence on long term survival. It is often used preoperatively to shrink the tumour and, with luck, render excision margins less critical. In addition, judicious chemotherapy may effectively palliate advanced head and neck cancers. It may, however, be difficult to ensure that the side effects of chemotherapy are not worse than the symptoms from the cancer.

Radiotherapy

Radiotherapy is important in the management of head and neck cancer and may be used as the sole intended treatment. For most small, localised tumours of the head and neck surgery and radiotherapy are equivalent in terms of cure and complications. The exceptions to this are the buccal sulcus, where surgery is to be preferred because of the risk of postradiation fibrosis producing trismus. Radiotherapy is the treatment of choice for most laryngeal tumours as the voice can usually be preserved.

Radiotherapy and surgery can be integrated in several ways. Radical radiotherapy (with curative intent) may be followed by salvage surgery for patients whose disease persists or recurs after irradiation. A standard course of radical radiotherapy for head and neck cancer comprises 60 to 65 Gy (6000-6500 rad) given in 30 to 35 fractions over six to seven weeks. A less protracted alternative is 50 to 55 Gy (5000-5500 rad) given in 15 fractions over three weeks.

Radiotherapy can be given before planned surgery in two ways: "flash" treatment (20 Gy (2000 rad) in four fractions in a week) or conventional preoperative treatment (40 Gy (4000 rad) in 20 fractions over four weeks). The conventional course allows the response of the tumour to be observed. If this has been exceptionally favourable the planned surgery can be abandoned and radiotherapy continued to a full radical dose. The main advantage of flash preoperative treatment is that surgery can follow immediately after the radiotherapy, there being no need to wait for the acute radiation reaction to settle.

Postoperative radiotherapy is indicated when doubt exists about a surgical excision margin or when there is overt recurrence after radical surgery. Preoperative and postoperative radiotherapy may be combined in the so called "sandwich" technique.

For certain histologies and certain sites fast neutrons may have some biological advantages over conventional x rays.

Head and neck cancer

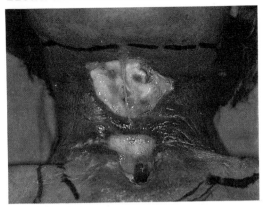

Cervical fistula.

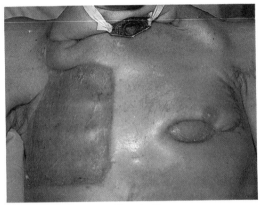

Repair using two pectoralis major flaps.

Elective surgical treatment of head and neck tumours requires complete excision of the tumour with a clear margin of normal tissue, which can be confirmed at the time of operation by frozen section histology. Reconstruction of the tissue deficit follows the principles of skin cover in other parts of the body—that is, primary closure should be used when possible. If there is no excess skin partial thickness grafts or, for cutaneous cancers, full thickness grafts should be employed. If, however, local tissues will not support a graft local flaps have to be employed, mobilising skin from areas where there is an excess—for example, in the nasolabial fold, in front of the ears, or around the eyes.

Surgery may be indicated also for palliation after other forms of treatment, particularly radiotherapy, have failed or caused complications. When radiotherapy has been used an endarteritis in the irradiated field produces problems with wound healing. In general, the area that has been irradiated requires radical excision, and distant flaps, usually based on the myocutaneous principle or in some cases free vascularised flaps, have to be employed to obtain wound cover. The main flaps used in the head and neck area are the pectoralis major, latissimus dorsi, and trapezius. The pectoralis major muscle flap allows skin to be mobilised from the chest based on the pectoralis muscle nourished from the thoracoacromial axis blood supply. The muscle and overlying skin can be transposed on this pedicle through 180° to cover a skin deficit in the lower third of the face and neck.

The advantages of surgery include the eradication of the primary cancer, an accurate histological assessment of the extent of the primary tumour, an accurate assessment of regional lymph node metastases, and immediate reconstruction. The disadvantages include the non-detection of occult extensions of the cancer cell at the periphery of the lesion, the loss of physiological function, and cosmetic disfigurement.

Cutaneous cancer

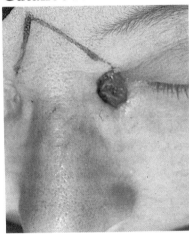
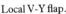
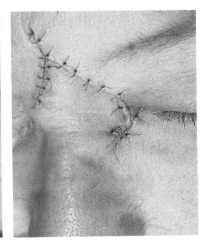

Local V-Y flap.

Surgical excision and plastic surgical repair of cutaneous cancer in the head and neck area have extremely high cure rates. Around the eyes, nose, and ears recurrence rates are, however, higher, reflecting a tendency to minimise mutilation and thereby compromise the adequacy of excision. There is also the possibility of field changes in surrounding skin associated with actinic damage. Despite this, surgery is in general preferred because cosmetically the results are usually superior to those of radiotherapy and any recurrence after radiotherapy in these difficult areas presents a major problem for reconstruction. The apex of the scalp also presents a major problem when major tissue excision has occurred as there are no local flaps available and free flaps therefore have to be used.

Intraoral carcinoma

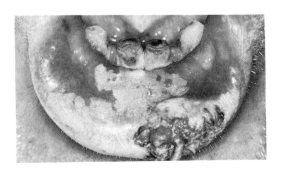

Roughly 1500 new cases of oral cancer present each year in England and Wales, 90% of which are squamous cell carcinomas. Formerly, there was an appreciable preponderance in men, but now there is an almost even distribution between the sexes in the south east of England. Though intraoral tumours may be treated by either radiotherapy or surgery, those adjacent to the buccal sulcus are best treated by surgery as radiotherapy may induce trismus. These tumours metastasise to the upper cervical lymph nodes and may directly invade into the mandible.

It is now apparent that resection of the mandible can be far more conservative even when the carcinoma has spread to the draining lymph nodes as the periosteum is an initial barrier to direct spread, and the lymphatic vessels themselves do not pass through the bone. Tumour

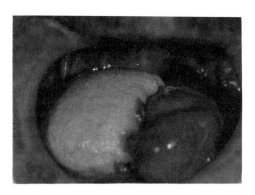

Radial forearm flap repairing extensive resection in the floor of mouth and tongue.

resection that includes bone, especially affecting the lower jaw, does not always require bony reconstruction. If, however, more than half the mandible is excised, and particularly if this is the anterior half, bony reconstruction is necessary. This is best achieved by a vascularised bone graft, especially if radiotherapy has been used previously. This can be achieved either by a radial forearm flap with hemiradius to reconstruct the anterior mandible or the iliac crest incorporated in a groin flap based on the deep circumflex iliac vessels, which can be used to reconstruct a complete hemimandible.

Pain associated with intraoral carcinoma may indicate perineural infiltration and carries a sinister prognosis. The reconstructive possibilities have been radically altered over the past 10 years. Whereas formerly the forehead flap was used to reconstruct the oral cavity, the recently introduced radial forearm flap now permits reconstruction without further mutilation in the head and neck area from local flaps such as the forehead.

Maxillary tumours

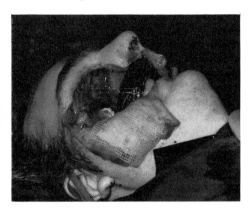

Maxillary tumours may be carcinomas arising from the upper alveolus or palate or may originate in the paranasal sinuses and invade downwards. They may also invade the orbital floor and extend into the base of the brain. Accurate preoperative assessment is vital. The maxilla may be approached surgically by turning a flap consisting of the upper lip and cheek laterally like a leaf of a book. The maxilla can be removed together with the orbit if necessary, and if there is extension to the base of the skull an anterior craniotomy may be performed for clearance above and below the base of the skull.

Reconstruction consists of a well fitting obturator to replace the bony loss with a skin graft to line the cheek. When surgery has extended to the base of the skull a skin flap is required to seal off the brain. This can be achieved either by an extended myocutaneous flap or by a free flap.

Regional lymph nodes

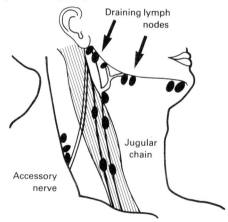

Once the tumour has spread to the regional nodes, and providing these nodes are mobile, surgical excision including all the cervical nodes in a block dissection is preferable to radiotherapy. If the nodes are fixed some form of combined treatment will be required.

The role of prophylactic block dissection of the clinically negative neck is controversial. There is no evidence that this improves the overall prognosis, but it may be indicated for some patients with large primary tumours.

Radical block dissection of the cervical nodes is associated with high morbidity, both functional and cosmetic. It causes limited abduction and pain in the shoulder and deformity because of loss of sternomastoid muscle. Functional block dissections have recently been introduced. The lymph nodes surrounding the internal jugular vein are removed, but the sternomastoid muscle and the accessory nerve supplying the trapezius muscle are preserved.

Prosthodontics

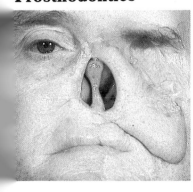

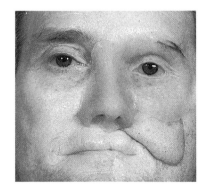

Although reconstructive techniques represent a major advance in the management of head and neck cancer in the past 15 years, the superb results that are now produced by the prosthesist in camouflaging tissue loss should not be forgotten. Often an artificial nose or an orbit with surrounding adnexa attached to a spectacle frame provides camouflage that cannot be approached by reconstructive surgery.

Head and neck cancer
Complications of treatment

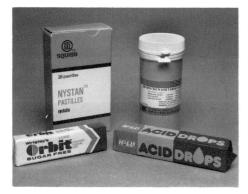

Oral lubricants.

Mucositis and stomatitis are inevitable complications of radiotherapy acute reactions. The severity varies with the dose, time, type, and fractionation of the radiotherapy. Patients should be advised to avoid alcohol, hot spicy food, and tobacco during treatment. Laryngeal oedema is a longer term complication; voice rest and humidified air will minimise discomfort. Patients should be told to seek immediate medical advice if stridor or respiratory difficulty develops. Swelling of the face and neck may occur during radiotherapy, particularly in patients who have had radical neck dissections. Patients should sleep with the head of the bed raised and avoid sleeping on the treated side.

When the salivary glands are within the treated area the saliva will become scant and tenacious. This effect may be temporary or permanent. Inevitably, loss of, and changes in, taste will occur. Sugarless chewing gum, acid or citrus sweets, or saliva substitutes (orex or xerolube) may help.

The dental management of patients undergoing radiotherapy is controversial. Formerly, routine complete dental clearance was advocated when the lower jaw was within the radiation field. Nowadays, a more conservative approach can be justified. Dental assessment before treatment and careful oral hygiene during and after treatment are essential. In this way, severe problems with caries and osteoradionecrosis of the mandible should be avoided.

Care of the tracheostomy

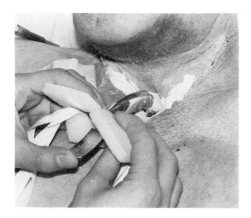

The airway should be kept free of secretions, and the patient must be encouraged to cough. It is essential to use a tracheostomy tube with an inner cannula for easy cleaning and an outer tube to keep the airway patent. The patient should be taught to clean the entire tube after its removal; a clean technique should be used rather than a sterile procedure.

Tenacious secretions of mucous crusting can be alleviated by placing several drops of sterile normal saline solution directly into the stoma to moisten the mucosa. The skin around the stoma should be washed with simple water and mild soap, and a thin layer of dimethicone cream or petroleum jelly should be applied around the stoma to protect the skin and decrease crusting. In cold weather extra bibs or stoma covers should be used to prevent cold air entering the stoma. If the tracheostomy is temporary the patient may be fitted with a speaking tracheostomy tube. After laryngectomy oesophageal speech can sometimes be learnt or the patient may resort to the use of an artificial larynx.

Care of the mouth and nutrition

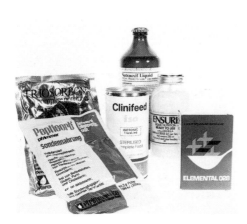

Irrigations are vital in keeping the operative area free from debris. Solutions of hydrogen peroxide or salt and soda are suitable. Halitosis is best avoided by cleaning the mouth with a soft toothbrush, toothpaste, and dental floss. Brushing of the tongue may be helpful.

Adequate nutritional intake is important, and patients will tolerate small, frequent meals. If feeding tubes are required commercial preparations are available for feeding. All feeding should begin and end with a little water to clean the nasogastric tube and maintain its patency. Some patients may complain of aspiration when swallowing; changing position during eating may alleviate this problem. Alcoholic patients are particularly susceptible to malnutrition during or after treatment and should therefore be carefully assessed and monitored.

THE HAND: CONGENITAL AND DEGENERATIVE DISEASES

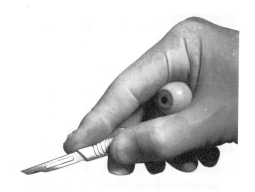

The hand is a highly specialised organ that has developed over thousands of years from the primitive fish pectoral fin. It is part of a multijoint system extending from the clavicle and scapula which allows a prodigious range of movement together with fine dexterity and also great strength. Its well developed sensory function results in it being described as the third eye.

Congenital hand abnormalities

Hand anomalies occur in about 1 per 700 live births. Some hand deformities are often associated with generalised syndromes—for example, Poland's syndrome, which includes a hypoplastic hand and the absence of or hypoplasia of the breast and underlying pectoral muscle on the same side.

Timing of surgery

There is no unanimity about the precise timing of surgery, although there is agreement that factors in favour of early surgery are: (*a*) very early surgery within 3 months of birth can be done on a thin hand; (*b*) the reconstructed part can be used early in development; and (*c*) psychologically it helps parents. Against early surgery are the facts that (*a*) the hand is small and often very fatty in the first year or two of life, (*b*) the bones are small and therefore postoperative immobilisation can be difficult, and (*c*) there is little cooperation from the patient.

All reconstructive surgery should be completed before the child goes to school, usually between the ages of 2 and 4 years, although policisation of an index finger for an absent thumb is often best performed far earlier. As with all hand surgery, it is important to remember that even though a child may have a severe abnormality there may be very little functional disability and in general cosmesis alone is not a reason to operate.

Syndactyly, one of the two most common congenital anomalies, is a failure of separation of the distally progressing finger elements. In simple cases it consists of only a skin bridge but in compound cases it affects the digital bones and joints. It is often associated with other anomalies. Bone union causes increasing deformity because of disproportionate growth, and the fingers should therefore be separated early. No matter how simple the syndactyly there is always a shortage of skin. This may be replaced by skin taken from either the groin or the instep of the foot. The dressings are usually left for two weeks, and then the patient will often need splints or a pressure garment during scar maturation.

Complete absence of the thumb is rare (though it was more prevalent when thalidomide was used), but it is important to treat it because the thumb contributes 45% of hand function. Policisation of the index finger, whereby it is shortened and transferred to the thumb is the treatment of choice. The interosseus muscles are used to construct thenar muscles. Advantages of this procedure are that an aesthetically pleasing new thumb is produced, which has good sensation and useful active opposition to the other fingers.

Classification

Failure of differentiation—for example, syndactyly
Arrest of development—for example, phocomelia
Congenital absence—for example, no thumb
Duplications—for example, extra digits
Overgrowth
Constriction bands
Generalised skeletal abnormality

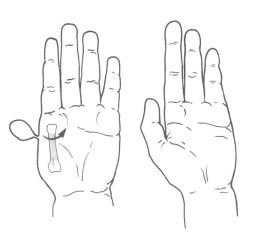

Excision of part of first metacarpal plus rotation.

The hand: congenital and degenerative diseases
Rheumatoid arthritis

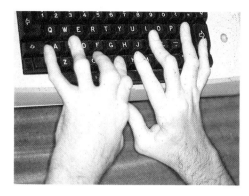

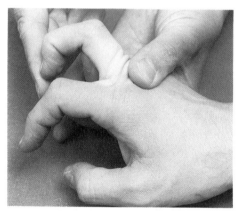

If the intrinsics are short the proximal interphalangeal joint cannot be flexed when the metacarpophalangeal joint is extended.

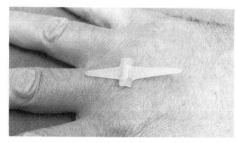

A Swanson arthroplasty.

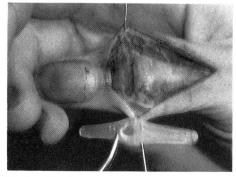

Harrison-Nicolle polypropylene peg.

Patients with rheumatoid arthritis are best managed in a combined clinic so that there is consultation between the rheumatologist, the hand surgeon, and the hand therapist. Many patients with severe chronic hand deformities are able to do most activities of daily living through trick or substitution motions, and thus preoperative assessment should be thorough and practical. The mere existence of a deformity is not an indication for surgery, and the aim should be to relieve pain, prevent further damage, and restore function. The patient must also realise that the operation will only interrupt a progressive disease and not cure it. Other joints in the body are often affected by the disease and there may be other medical conditions to consider. A patient who is being considered for surgery must be able to cooperate, particularly in the rehabilitation programme, if he is to get the best from the surgery.

Surgery is based on five procedures:

Joint synovectomy—In rheumatoid arthritis the synovium proliferates, causing necrosis of the joint cartilage, and also stretches the supporting structures—the collateral ligaments—and eventually causes their destruction. Synovectomy should be undertaken before these two processes become apparent, and in general it is usually performed too late. Most hand surgeons believe that some benefit is derived from synovectomy, which can never be complete, but there is little proof of this as controls are extremely difficult because of the progressive nature of the disease. Undoubtedly it provides good pain relief with minimal risk of functional loss.

Tenosynovectomy—Synovial proliferation also occurs in the tendon sheaths on the dorsal and volar aspects of the wrist and the flexor tendon sheaths of the fingers. This can compress the median nerve at the wrist and produce limited painful movement, locking of the fingers on flexion, or tendon rupture. Tenosynovectomy at the wrist will relieve local symptoms, but radical tenosynovectomy of the flexor tendon sheaths may have a high morbidity.

Tendon surgery—Rupture of the tendons, particularly the extensor tendons of the thumb, ring, and little fingers, occurs through their attrition as they glide over the dorsum of the wrist. The most common form of repair is to suture the distal divided tendon to an adjacent, intact tendon. If the extensor tendon in the thumb is ruptured then one of the two extensor tendons in the index finger is transferred. Boutonnière and Swan neck deformities are both common in rheumatoid arthritis. Boutonnière deformity is caused by rupture or an attenuation of the central slip of the extensor tendon inserting into the middle phalanx. Swan neck deformity is usually associated with intrinsic muscle tightness, which alters the balance of the complicated extensor tendon mechanism. Surgery for these two conditions depends on the underlying cause, and the results may be disappointing.

Arthroplasty—Despite an increasing awareness of the factors leading to finger and thumb deformities many patients ultimately develop joint subluxation and dislocation. Despite horrendous deformities in the hand, there may, however, be little incapacity. Joint prostheses may be inserted into the metocarpophalangeal joint and more rarely the proximal interphalangeal joint. Alignment of the finger is always improved by a successful arthroplasty operation, as is joint stability, but the actual movement through the metacarpophalangeal joint may not be improved. For painful disease at the wrist, especially where the ulnar styloid has become subluxed, ulnar styloidectomy can provide great symptomatic relief in most cases.

Arthrodesis—Despite improved artificial joints there continues to be an important place in rheumatoid surgery for joint fusion. Fusion is thought to be the best way to correct many of the advanced deformities and is particularly good in restoring the pinch stability of the thumb and index and middle fingers. Arthrodesis also is successful for severe disease at the wrist, which is of great importance as it is the key to the function of all the other joints in the hand. The wrist should be immobilised in a neutral position; the use of intramedullary fixation prevents the need for prolonged plaster immobilisation. Arthrodesis of the interphalangeal joints using a Harrison silastic peg, which can be straight or angled, is quick and simple.

Osteoarthritis

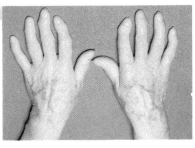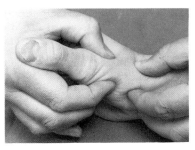

Grinding the thumb metacarpal on the trapezium (right) causes pain in a diseased joint.

The incidence of osteoarthritis is high. The cause remains unknown, but there is an interplay of genetic and mechanical factors leading to biomechanical alterations in the cartilage. Disabling osteoarthritis of the hand is often misdiagnosed. Many patients respond well to simple physical and medical therapy and by moderating their activities. Patients with destructive joint disease in the digits can have excellent results with arthrodesis and implant arthroplasty for the basal joint of the thumb, which are the most common joints affected.

Dupuytren's disease

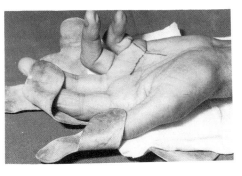

Dupuytren's disease is thought to be a genetic abnormality caused by a single dominant gene. The disease originated in the Celtic races of northern Europe and has been disseminated by migration to Australia and North America. Its incidence in Scotland is about 25% in men over 65 years of age. It is much more common in patients with epilepsy.

Treatment

Fifty per cent of patients followed up for more than five years will show recurrence or extension of the disease, but it is not possible to predict which patients these will be, and there is an appreciable morbidity from radical surgery. The surgeon should plan operations appropriate to the patient's age, general health, extent of the disease, and rate of progression. Hueston suggests that if the patient can not place his hand and fingers flat on a table then surgery is advisable. It is always possible to correct contracture of the metacarpophalangeal joint but it is not always possible to correct flexion at the proximal interphalangeal joint, especially if it has been present for any length of time. The aim of treatment should be to control the disease and at the same time retain as much hand function as possible.

Four operations are available:

Fasciotomy—A single band of fascia is divided either blindly subcutaneously or after more formal dissection. In the old patient this operation has a lot to offer especially for disease in the palm of the hand.

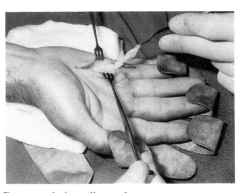

Dupuytren's tissue dissected.

Fasciectomy—Radical fasciectomy, especially in the palm of the hand, is no longer advocated. In general a limited fasciectomy is performed in the palm and this may be extended into the fingers, where a more extensive dissection may be required. Skin can be closed either by direct suture or, if a transverse incision is made, by a skin graft, or it may be left open.

Open palm technique of McCash—A transverse incision is made and if there is a relative shortage of skin the hand can be splinted and the fingers extended, leaving a skin deficit in the hand. This is left to heal spontaneously, within four to six weeks. The skin incision heals, leaving a linear scar and the fingers in an extended position.

Fasciectomy and skin graft—This procedure is based on the observation that Dupuytren's disease does not usually recur beneath a full thickness skin graft. This technique may be reserved for recurrent disease or for patients with a strong Dupuytren's diathysis in whom the likelihood of recurrence is high.

Postoperative complications

The overall complication rate is high (20%) and includes haematoma, skin necrosis, and infection, which are a related triad and usually follow extensive operations in the palm, especially where there has been tight skin closure. This sequence may precipitate reflex sympathetic dystrophy, which occurs in up to 3% of operations and is more common in women. More seriously, damage to digital nerves or loss of a finger may also occur.

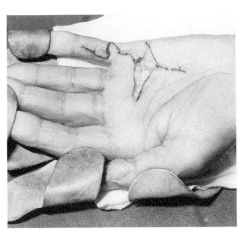

Open palm technique of McCash.

The hand: congenital and degenerative diseases
Ganglion

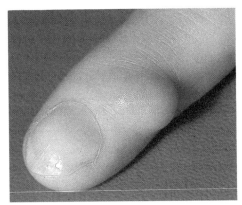

Ganglion arising from distal interphalangeal joint.

The most common hand tumour presents usually as a cystic swelling. The peak incidence is in the young adult. The most common sites of presentation are: (*a*) next to the wrist either on the volar aspect, usually near the radial artery where it may communicate with the radial carpal, or on the inferior radial lunar joint; (*b*) on the dorsal aspect of the wrist commonly arising from the scapholunate or mid carpal joint, where it may give rise to pain and weakness of the wrist; (*c*) at the base of the finger, arising from the proximal end of the digital flexor tendon sheath; and (*d*) arising from the distal interphalangeal joint on the dorsal aspect adjacent to the nail bed.

Treatment

Up to half of all ganglia disappear spontaneously. Rupture by firm pressure or banging with a family bible has a high recurrence rate, as does aspiration and injection of cortisone. Surgical excision is indicated for those lesions causing discomfort, pain, or nerve compression. The success of the operation depends on successful dissection of the communication down to the point of origin from a joint or synovial sheath. The operation should therefore be done under a tourniquet with either regional or general anaesthesia and the incisions should be large enough to allow adequate surgical exposure of the structures.

Carpal tunnel syndrome

Symptoms

Numbness in distribution of median nerve to thumb and fingers
Pain severest at night, relieved by opening and closing fingers
Pain on acutely flexing wrist
Clumsiness of hand
Muscle wasting at thenar eminence
Sensory disturbance
Positive Tennel sign at wrist

Causes

Developmental
  Neurofibromatosis
  Anomalous intrinsic or extrinsic muscles
  Persistently large median artery
Traumatic
  Colles fracture
  Indirect damage—for example, severe trauma to hand resulting in oedema
Inflammatory
  Rheumatoid arthritis
Tumour
  Ganglion or lipoma
Endocrine
  Pregnancy or myxoedema

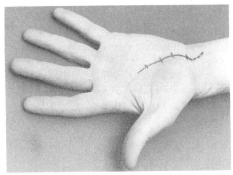

Line of surgical incision.

Carpal tunnel syndrome results from compression of the median nerve within the carpal tunnel. It can occur in adults of any age but usually occurs in those aged 30-60 years. It is rare in children, in whom it is usually associated with neurofibromatosis. It is five times more common in women than in men and occurs more often in the dominant hand; however, both hands are often affected. In men the disease is unusual but may be associated with vibrating tools.

On the flexor aspect of the wrist there are three canals: on the radial side that for the flexor carpi radialis tendon, on the ulnar side Guyon's tunnel, where the ulnar artery and nerve lie, and in between the carpal tunnel, through which 10 structures pass, including most superficially the median nerve. Any component or content of the carpal tunnel which increases in size will compress the nerve. A pressure of 30 mm Hg is enough to reduce the intraneural vascular blood flow.

Treatment

Conservative treatment in mild symptomatic cases and in pregnancy consists of splintage, restricting activity of the hand, corticosteroid injections into the canal, and diuretics in pregnancy. Conservative treatment may also include vitamin B_6 100-200 mg daily for two to 12 weeks.

About 40% of patients need surgical treatment carried out under regional block or general anaesthesia with tourniquet. The carpal ligament should not be divided blindly through a very proximal incision, but the incision should be made on the ulnar aspect on the thenar crease. This allows the carpal ligament to be divided under direct vision and prevents damage to an abnormally situated thenar motor branch. After operation there may be weakness of the wrist and hand for several months and the scar may be associated with painful neuromas. In a very few cases there may be a persistent carpal tunnel syndrome which is due to incomplete divison of the flexor retinaculum or due to fibrosis around or in the median nerve.

Carpal tunnel decompression totally relieves symptoms in half the cases, but in about 10% there is little improvement.

THE HAND: TRAUMA

Infections

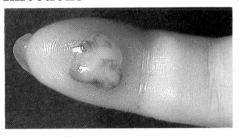

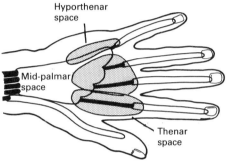

Hyporthenar space

Mid-palmar space

Thenar space

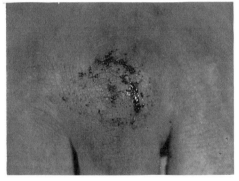

The ultimate aim in managing injuries and infections of the hand is to produce a pain free, stable, and mobile hand.

Paronconychia (whitlow) is an acute or chronic infection around the nail. Pus initially accumulates between the cuticle and the nail matrix. Treatment includes draining the abscess and splinting and raising the hand. The usual organism is a staphylococcus. Chronic paronconychia is usually caused by a combination of low grade staphylococcal and candidal infection. If the lesion is not cured by appropriate chemotherapy then excision of the adjacent nail may help.

Infection of the pulp space (felon) is often extremely painful because the fibrous septa limits the spread of any pus. The increase in pressure can cause thrombosis of the small distal digital vessels and in a chronic case can lead to avascular necrosis of the distal phalanx, beyond the epiphyseal plate.

Web space infection—The palmar space, the thenar space, and the flexor tendon sheaths may become infected. Again treatment depends on drainage and antistaphylococcal antibiotics. In suppurative tenosynovitis the finger becomes swollen and sausage like and is held in the flexed position; movement causes extreme pain. The tendon sheath may have to be irrigated with solution of benzylpenicillin.

Human bites are usually sustained in fights when a blow to the opponent's teeth causes a laceration over the dorsum of the metocarpopharyngeal joint. The injury is usually compound, affecting the skin, the underlying extensor tendon, and the joint cavity. The wound may be contaminated by foreign bodies, especially fragments of broken teeth. These injuries are renowned for their initial trivial appearance belying their severity. This may become manifest only when the wound has failed to heal after many weeks and with the development of a septic arthritis. The wound should be explored and wound swabs taken for aerobic and anaerobic culture. The wound should then be carefully debrided and the hand must be raised and splinted. Delayed repair of structures is best, together with the use of both antistaphylococcal and antianaerobic chemotherapy (metronidazole).

Foreign bodies

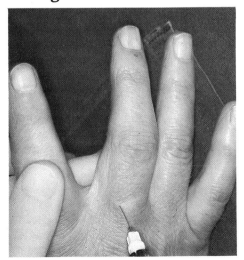

Foreign bodies are common in injuries to the hand. These may present acutely or through chronic infection. In the case of non-irritant foreign bodies such as broken ends of needles, flakes of steel from grinding machines, and small fragments of glass, a "wait and observe" policy can be advocated, especially if the fragments lie deep in the hand. Provided the foreign body is small it causes little problem and becomes sealed off by a fibrous capsule. This makes it easier to locate if it does go on to cause trouble. Irritant foreign bodies, in particular wooden splinters, rose thorns, cacti, and sea urchins' spines, are best explored at the time of presentation, before frank abscesses develop. Radiographs taken in two planes with a marker attached to the skin may help to locate radio-opaque foreign bodies.

Digital nerve block. Needle inserted through dorsal aspect and advanced until it is felt under the skin on the palmar aspect. Plain lignocaine is then injected as the needle is withdrawn along its whole course.

The hand: trauma

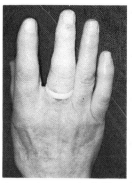 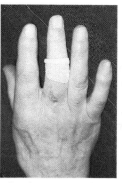 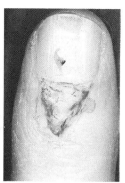

Exploration should be undertaken under the very best of surgical conditions with good lighting, a bloodless field provided by a tourniquet, and good anaesthesia by either local digital nerve block, regional block, or general anaesthesia.

A tourniquet can be fashioned using the amputated finger of a sterile glove.

Nail injuries

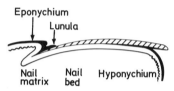

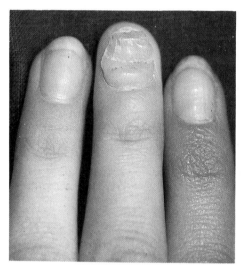

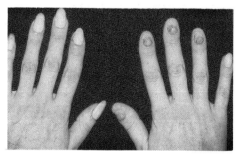

The nail is a keratinised, epidermal skin appendage. It supports the terminal pulp of the finger and is therefore important in helping sensation and grip. It also has an aesthetic property and may occasionally have a combative function. Nails grow at about 1 mm a week, more rapidly in the hand than in the foot, in the young, in the middle finger, and in the dominant hand.

A blunt crush injury to the tip of the finger can produce a closed injury and subungual haematoma. The haematoma is under high pressure and is therefore very painful. Initial treatment by elevation and cold compresses can help, but trephining the nail with the end of a heated paper clip produces instantaneous relief.

A more severe injury may avulse the nail either partially or completely. Any part of the nail can become dislocated but usually the proximal nail becomes sprung from underneath the nail bed fold. In more severe injuries the nail can be completely detached with or without damage to the underlying matrix or nail bed, and there may be an accompanying phalangeal fracture. If the nail bed is undamaged the nail will regenerate, and so long as no adhesions occur between the lunula and the nail bed there will be no surface irregularities in this new nail. Adhesions are best prevented by replacing the avulsed nail in its exact position, using it both as a splint to the nail matrix and as a dressing to the nail bed. Injuries to the nail bed are important, since any surface irregularity will lead to a new nail being deformed. Lacerations should be accurately repaired using magnification. Any tissue loss should be replaced with a partial thickness skin graft.

Late deformities of the nail are extremely difficult to treat both cosmetically and functionally. Many patients may best be served cosmetically by having their nail removed and using an artificial nail. More modern microvascular techniques allow nails and nail beds to be transferred from the toes to the hand using the dorsalis pedis artery and vein. This is, of course, a surgical tour de force.

Pulp tip injuries

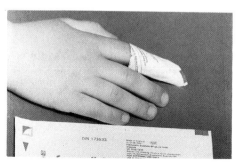

Injuries to the finger tip can be either simple lacerations, guillotine amputations, or crush injuries producing a more extensive ragged bursting type of injury. On initial examination the clinician should try to assess the amount of skin loss, whether there is exposed bone, and the viability of the remaining skin. In young children most injuries can be treated conservatively even when there is extensive skin loss and exposed bone, as the finger tips in this age group have remarkable abilities to heal, and even possibly regenerate. Skin that is present and viable should be replaced in the correct position; pieces of skin can be retained with Steristrips, but these must not be placed circumferentially around the finger. The best splintage and dressing is provided by the corner of the aluminium foil packet which is used to package petroleum jelly gauze dressings.

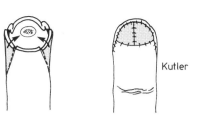
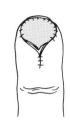

Kutler

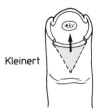

Kleinert

In an adult the type of repair should depend on the type of injury, the finger affected, the age and occupation of the patient, and the manual dexterity that he requires. Where there is pure skin loss a partial thickness skin graft is the simplest method of coverage; this will eventually contract leaving a scarred tip to the finger. If this provides unsuitable cover a later reconstruction with local flaps can be performed. For some patients, particularly those for whom cosmesis is important, the finger length can be maintained by the use of local flaps. These are best used where there are straight or dorsally angled amputations. In other cases cross finger or thenar flaps may be used but the disadvantages of these types of repair are the scars produced on other fingers and the three weeks' immobilisation, which may produce stiffness in both the injured finger and other joints of the hand. In a manual worker with thick fingers who does not require fine manual dexterity and where there is exposed bone the simplest procedure may be to nibble back the exposed bone and perform a distal amputation. This usually provides the quickest form of healing and thus gets the patient back to work in the shortest possible time.

Joint injury

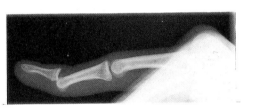

Joint injuries are common, often sustained during fights or sporting activities. The patient presents with a swollen tender finger joint. If there is a nearly complete full range of active movement with no instability then there is probably no serious injury. Such a "sprain" may extend as far as a partial tear of the collateral ligament. Such minor injuries often remain painful for six months, swollen for two years, and cause considerable inconvenience, but they usually settle without any specific treatment. The major point of management is early mobilisation to avoid joint stiffness. When there is limited or abnormal movement the lesion is more sinister, and anteroposterior and true lateral radiographs should be taken of the joint. Any subluxation or dislocation should be reduced. If it is not easily reduced by manipulation then an open reduction should be performed as this usually indicates soft tissue interference with the reduction. When there has been a complete tear of the collateral ligament or volar plate, as often indicated by a flake fracture on the x ray film, open reduction and fixation are required.

Mallet finger injuries

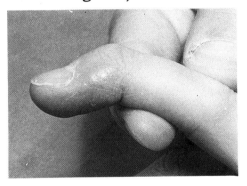

Mallet injuries are a disruption of the distal part of the extensor mechanism of the finger, distal to the interphalangeal joint. Only the tendon may have been ruptured, but many of these injuries also include avulsion of a small fragment of bone at the insertion. When there is no associated fracture splintage of the extended finger for six weeks is sufficient. If there is a large fragment of bone attached to the ruptured tendon, and especially if more than a third of the joint surface is affected, open reduction and fixation should be performed. It is important that the patient retains good flexion at the interphalangeal joint, and this should not be compromised by trying to gain a complete range of extension.

Management of lacerations

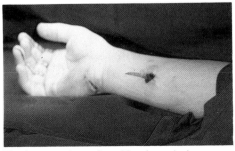

Nowhere is it more important that an accurate history and careful and thorough examination should be undertaken than with lacerations, for primary repair offers the best results to most such injuries. Inappropriate treatment or missed injuries to deeper structures lying beneath a trivial skin wound can lead to some patients requiring extensive secondary surgery. In some cases the end result is a useless, painful, stiff finger, hand, or arm—with crippling consequences. Examination of such an injury should follow the time honoured orthopaedic system of taking a history and then looking, feeling, and moving.

The dangerous laceration with a glass spicule.

The hand: trauma

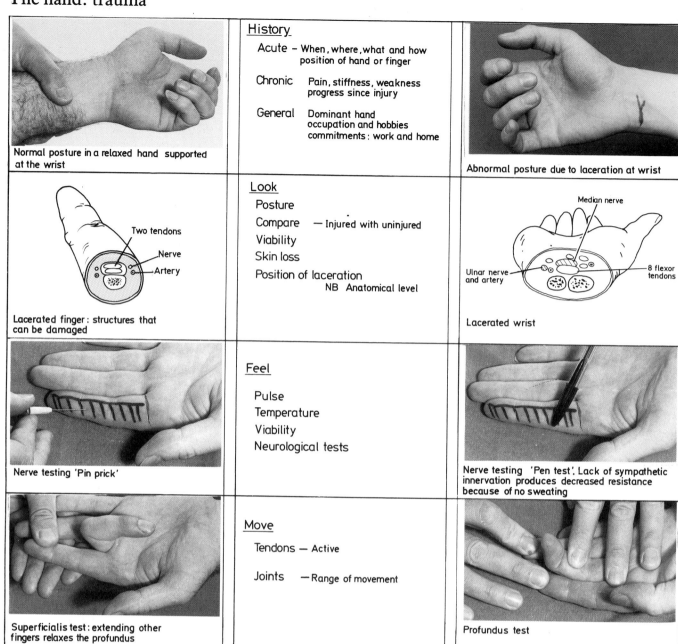

Normal posture in a relaxed hand supported at the wrist

History

Acute – When, where, what and how position of hand or finger

Chronic — Pain, stiffness, weakness progress since injury

General — Dominant hand occupation and hobbies commitments: work and home

Abnormal posture due to laceration at wrist

Look

Posture

Compare — Injured with uninjured

Viability

Skin loss

Position of laceration
NB Anatomical level

Lacerated finger: structures that can be damaged

Two tendons
Nerve
Artery

Lacerated wrist

Median nerve
Ulnar nerve and artery
8 flexor tendons

Feel

Pulse

Temperature

Viability

Neurological tests

Nerve testing 'Pin prick'

Nerve testing 'Pen test'. Lack of sympathetic innervation produces decreased resistance because of no sweating

Move

Tendons — Active

Joints — Range of movement

Superficialis test: extending other fingers relaxes the profundus

Profundus test

Fractures of the hand

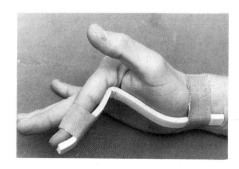

As with other fractures, treatment of fractures of the hand depends on reduction, retention, and rehabilitation. Three groups can be identified.

The minimally displaced but stable fracture may be rested for a few days to allow the swelling to settle and the pain to subside. This then allows the adjacent joints to be mobilised within a few days, which is important to prevent stiffness. Swelling, which has been called the cement of the hand, can be reduced by keeping the hand raised in a high sling and elevating it on pillows by the side of the bed at night. Seventy per cent of fractured phalanges can be mobilised early.

Most unstable fractures can be treated by reduction and splintage in the correct position, which is with the metocarpophalangeal joint flexed and the interphalangeal joint in extension. Splintage can be achieved by strapping to the adjacent finger, allowing a dynamic form of support, or by using an external metal Zimmer splint, or plaster of Paris front slab. It is important to check the position of the tips of the fingers for malrotation. Twenty five per cent of fractured phalanges require such treatment.

A minority of unstable fractures or failed closed reductions require internal fixation. This may also be necessary in displaced fractures close to a joint, multiple fractures, or where the finger has been replanted. However, this type of management accounts for only about five per cent of cases.

Flexor tendon injuries

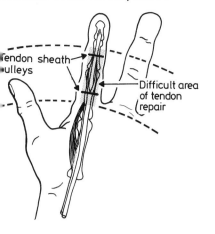

The flexor tendons pass through the carpal tunnel and both a superficial and a profundus tendon supply each finger. For most of the length of the finger the two tendons lie next to each other in a flexor tendon sheath. Injuries to these tendons in the finger have until recently been associated with a very bad prognosis and in the past tendons were not repaired primarily: management was by a delayed tendon graft. Modern methods of tendon repair, in which both tendons are repaired at the time of injury with careful postoperative supervision using dynamic traction, provide far better results than either delayed repair or tendon grafting. Tendon repair is performed under tourniquet and the incisions need to be extended to oppose the two ends of the tendon. The ends of the divided tendon should be handled as atraumatically as possible. The flexor tendon sheath must be repaired at the same time, as must the thickenings in the flexor tendon sheath which act as pulleys and keep the tendon adjacent to the phalanges.

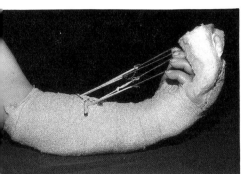

After operation the hand is raised and set in dynamic splintage. This comprises a protective back slab plaster with the wrist and the fingers flexed on a tight elastic band. Active extension allows the finger to be straightened but it is then returned to the flexed position by the pull of the elastic band. This protected movement should be maintained for six weeks, after which the patient should be referred for rehabilitation.

Repair of nerves

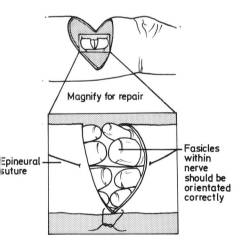

The repair of nerves remains a major problem in hand surgery. The most important factor other than the amount of damage at the division is the age of the patient. Young patients obtain good results, but in older patients, no matter how accurate the repair, the results will generally be disappointing. The best results are undoubtedly attained by primary repair of the nerve, the use of magnification, avoidance of any tension, and the provision of a well vascularised bed.

Four weeks' immobilisation is then usually necessary until the two ends are well joined. When major nerves are divided it is important that the patient realises that it will take many months before the nerves regenerate and that the results go on improving up to a year or more and may further be helped by sensory re-education.

Neuroma, causalgia, and reflex sympathetic dystrophy

When a nerve is divided the proximal fibres first degenerate and then regenerate, producing a large sprouting mass from the proximal end of the nerve. If these new nerve fibres fail to grow up the distal myelin sheath they eventually lead to formation of a neuroma. Such damage to a nerve may produce a range of symptoms ranging from a localised neuroma to, at its extreme, a painful, swollen, stiff hand with loss of hair, changes in the nail, and thinning or atrophy of the skin. Alternatively, the hand may be affected by hyperpathia, in which light touch causes severe pain, although there may be little associated sensory or motor loss.

Treatment consists of: (*a*) rehabilitation; (*b*) electrical counterstimulation, which decreases the ectopic generator firing; and (*c*) sympathetic block using guanethidine, which decreases the local noradrenaline concentration. Surgery has little part to play except in an unrepaired divided nerve. Simple resection of the neuroma rarely helps; neither do local blocks using phenol and alcohol.

The hand: trauma
Rehabilitation

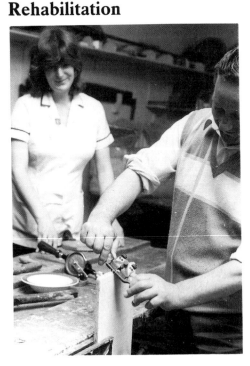

Two major factors determine the outcome of most hand surgery: firstly, the character of the patient, his willingness and enthusiasm to cooperate, withstand local pain and discomfort, and work diligently at rehabilitation; and, secondly, the provision of a properly manned occupational therapy and rehabilitation service. An occupational therapy unit must include a person who can attend the hand clinic regularly to provide assessment of hand function both before and after operation. This evaluation includes work and domestic environments and also assesses the range of movements in individual joints and the strength of various grips, etc. The facilities offered by the unit should include wax baths, an ice machine, ultrasound, and the ability to make customised splints. Once the initial surgery has been undertaken and the wounds have healed the patient should then progress to a home orientated unit; and there should be a workshop with the ability to adapt implements to preserve a patient's independence both at work and at home. After nerve repairs sensory retraining is important. This includes the recognising of shapes and textures of various fabrics and materials.